Optometric Management of Reading Dysfunction

Optometric Management of Reading Dysfunction

John R. Griffin, M. Opt., O.D., M.S.Ed.
Professor of Optometry, Department of Clinical Science,
Southern California College of Optometry, Fullerton

Garth N. Christenson, O.D., M.S.Ed.
Christenson Vision Care, Ltd., Hudson, Wisconsin;
Optometric Consultant, Chance to Grow/New Visions School,
Minneapolis, Minnesota

Michael D. Wesson, O.D., M.S.
Clinical Associate Professor of Optometry, University of Alabama at
Birmingham, School of Optometry, Birmingham

Graham B. Erickson, O.D.
Assistant Professor of Optometry, Department of Clinical Science,
Southern California College of Optometry, Fullerton

Butterworth–Heinemann
Boston   Oxford   Johannesburg   Melbourne   New Delhi   Singapore

Every effort has been made to ensure that the drug dosage schedules within this text are accurate and conform to standards accepted at time of publication. However, as treatment recommendations vary in the light of continuing research and clinical experience, the reader is advised to verify drug dosage schedules herein with information found on product information sheets. This is especially true in cases of new or infrequently used drugs.

 Recognizing the importance of preserving what has been written, Butterworth–Heinemann prints its books on acid-free paper whenever possible.

Library of Congress Cataloging-in-Publication Data

Optometric management of reading dysfunction / John R. Griffin . . . [et al.].
    p.   cm.
    Includes bibliographical references and index.
    ISBN 0-7506-9516-1
    1. Dyslexia—Treatment. 2. Reading disability—Treatment.
  3. Optometry. 4. Visual therapy.   I. Griffin, John R., 1934-
    [DNLM: 1. Dyslexia—therapy. 2. Perceptual Disorders—therapy.
    3. Visual Perception—physiology. 4. Vision Disorders—therapy.
  WL 340.6 062 1996]
  RJ61.068   1996
  616.85'5306—dc20
  DNLM/DLC
  for Library of Congress   96-43032
                                    CIP

British Library Cataloguing-in-Publication Data
A catalogue record for this book is available from the British Library.

The publisher offers special discounts on bulk orders of this book.
For information, please contact:

Manager of Special Sales
Butterworth–Heinemann
313 Washington Street
Newton, MA 02158-1626
Tel: 617-928-2500
Fax: 617-928-2620

For information on all medical publications available, contact our World Wide Web home page at: http://www.bh.com/med

10 9 8 7 6 5 4 3 2 1

Printed in the United States of America

Contents

Preface

This book is written to assist optometrists in the management of patients with reading dysfunction (RD). Other professionals of the multidisciplinary team, however, may find this information useful.

Confusion about the role of vision and the reading process has abounded since the introduction of the term *dyslexia* by eye care practitioners in the late 1800s. The purpose of this book is to provide the optometrist with information about the theory, testing, and management of RD, with an emphasis on vision-related etiologies. Discussions focus on a unifying model that is clinically applicable and reliable for both primary eye care practitioners and those who specialize in vision therapy. We also hope that the scientific principles in this text will be shared with educators to stimulate the use of appropriate multisensory structured-language teaching in schools. An understanding, by optometrists, educators, and other concerned professionals, of the relation of RD to dyslexia and vision problems will facilitate this needed intervention in schools.

Part I begins with a theoretic discussion of the causes of general and specific RD. The term *reading dysfunction* is also referred to as reading disability, reading disorder, reading difficulty, and reading problems, and encompasses both general and specific problems in reading. Discussion of language development from spoken to written language proficiency is presented. Following this, a comprehensive model is developed for dyslexia, a coding problem, which is specific RD. Although dyslexia has had many different meanings to practitioners, this book presents an operational definition based on well-founded neurologic and behavioral principles. A model is presented for the clinical diagnosis and treatment of individuals with RD, whether dyslexic or nondyslexic.

Part II discusses the physical and physiologic processes involved in reading. The role of low-level visual information processing (e.g., magnocellular pathway) is discussed in light of recent research on the spatial and temporal nature of reading. The role of higher levels of visual information processing (e.g., visual-perceptual-motor processing) is also discussed, in addition to auditory perception.

Part III covers clinical testing procedures for various sensory, motor, and perceptual vision problems that may result in general RD. Differential diagnosis of specific RD leads to the identification of the several types of dyslexia; appropriate tests are presented.

Part IV presents therapy methods for RD. Optometric vision therapy for related vision problems is discussed in detail. A multidisciplinary approach to management emphasizes educational therapy. Results of therapy are discussed, and case studies illustrate management options for various types of RD.

We thank the following individuals for their help in making this volume possible: Barbara Murphy and Karen Oberheim of Butterworth–Heinemann; Patricia Carlson, Judy Badstuebner, Patricia Humpres, Judy Higgins, Albert Garcia, Drs. Richard Hopping, Morris Berman, and Eric Borsting of the Southern California College of Optometry; Drs. Bradford Wild, Robert Kleinstein, Clyde Oyster, and Arol Augsberger of the University of Alabama at Birmingham, School of Optometry; Dr. Arthur Dahle of the Civitan International Research Center at the University of Alabama at Birmingham and Dr. T. Shroeder of Indiana University; and Sandra Romsos, R.N., Dr. Dina Hababa Erickson, Kirsten Griffin, R.N., and Mary Lou Christenson for help in manuscript preparation.

J.R.G.
G.N.C.
M.D.W.
G.B.E.

Optometric Management of Reading Dysfunction

I. Identifying Reading Dysfunction

1 General and Specific Reading Dysfunction

Learning disabilities, including those related to vision, encompass many more problems than reading dysfunction (RD). An individual with RD is one whose achievement in reading is significantly below expectancy. The term *dysfunction* is preferable to other descriptors, such as *disability* and *disorder*, which may imply intractability, or *difficulties* and *problems*, which are prognostically vague. Many of the vision problems related to RD can be eliminated completely with direct optometric intervention.[1] Some forms of RD, however, can be only partially improved with optometric intervention. Other forms can be identified by the optometrist, but their treatment depends mainly on educational therapy and intervention by other professionals.

Necessity of Literacy

Recognition of RD and its causes is crucial, now more than ever, because rapid advancements in the technologic evolution of our global society increasingly require workers with good reading skills. Countries with high-level technology at their disposal have been displacing functionally illiterate workers from the traditional workplace (functional illiteracy is usually defined as reading below the sixth-grade level). Workers in industrial jobs of an essentially nonreading nature, such as manual assembly-line jobs, are being replaced by automation and robotic manufacturing. Even jobs that used to require no great literacy have changed: The frustrated parents of a child with RD who say, "If he can't do anything else, he can drive a truck," are not aware that this is no longer such a clear-cut option. Interstate truck drivers in the United States are required to read detailed instructions, rules, and regulations, and must undergo vocational training and certification before being hired.[2] Functional illiteracy can no longer be tolerated in our increasingly complex society. Illiteracy adversely affects an individual's quality of life in school, work, and play.

Early identification and management of RD is essential for the future development of human potential in our rapidly changing society, and the optometrist has a key role to play in the process.

Causes of Reading Dysfunction

Vision and visual information processing problems (see Chapter 6) are associated with *general* RD.[3–6] We have seen optometric intervention assist children, teenagers, and adults to become better readers. On the other hand, successful vision therapy (as measured by improvement in visual skills) does not always eliminate RD, particularly in cases of dyslexia.

Nonvisual causes of RD should also be identified for referral to other professionals of the management team. This team may consist of educators, psychologists, physicians, and other professionals concerned with RD. For example, lack of motivation (relating to affect regulation), a concern for psychologists and trained counselors, may be a major factor in preventing an individual's reading progress. RD may also result from severe allergies, for which medical treatment may be warranted.

We classify RD as either *nonspecific* (general) or *specific* (dyslexic). General reading problems have many etiologies, which may exist in isolation or in combination. Christenson et al.[7] listed several of these causes of general RD, shown in Table 1.1.

A specific reading problem can be considered synonymous with the term *dyslexia*. Dyslexia, as we and others[7–13] define it, is a *coding* problem involving written language that results in poor reading, spelling, and writing. Dyslexia is not a primary comprehension problem, but reading comprehension is secondarily affected if decoding (i.e., recognition) of words is poor. If an individual cannot decode many of the important words in a passage, reading comprehension of that passage is consequently poor. The coding problem of dyslexia is thought to be due to a neurologic dysfunction or a differential brain function (cognitive strengths and weaknesses peculiar to each individual).[14] We agree with the following general statement by the Research Committee of the Orton Dyslexia Society[15]:

TABLE 1.1   Major Causes of General Reading Dysfunction

Low intelligence (e.g., full-scale IQ <80 on the Wechsler Intelligence Scale for Children–Revised)
Educational deprivation (e.g., child who does not attend school regularly)
Sociocultural deprivation or differences (e.g., English is child's second language)
Primary emotional or mental health problems (e.g., schizophrenia)
Vision problems (e.g., high uncorrected hyperopic astigmatism)
Auditory problems (e.g., poor auditory discrimination)
Sensory-integration problems (e.g., poor auditory-visual integrative skills)
Attentional problems (e.g., attention-deficit hyperactivity disorder)
Other problems as well as many possible unknown causes (e.g., allergies affecting an individual's ability to stay on task, poor motivation, poor nutrition, speech problems, undetected physical and mental health problems)

> *Dyslexia is one of several distinct learning disabilities. It is a specific language-based disorder of constitutional origin characterized by difficulties in single word decoding, usually reflecting insufficient phonological processing abilities. These difficulties in single word decoding are often unexpected in relation to age and other cognitive and academic abilities; they are not the result of generalized developmental disability or sensory impairment. Dyslexia is manifested by variable difficulty with different forms of language, often including, in addition to problems reading, a conspicuous problem with acquiring proficiency in writing and spelling.*

Dyslexia should be considered as a separate entity; it causes specific decoding and encoding patterns that are consistently evident in the affected individual. Although the label of *dyslexia* is not without controversy, we prefer this diagnostic term to other possible terms because it is widely used and recognized. In the past, the term *dyslexia* has had different meanings to many clinicians, leading to considerable confusion. We present an operational definition later in this book (see Chapters 3 and 10 for further discussion of dyslexia).

Dyslexia should not be confused with factors that cause general problems in reading, writing, and spelling (see Table 1.1). Of these general factors, low intelligence is probably the most easily understood cause. A child with significantly reduced mental ability demonstrates generally poor reading skills due to poor comprehension, even if decoding skills are relatively good. Other areas of learning, such as mathematics, are also affected by a low IQ. Dyslexia, on the other hand, affects the individual's ability to decode words but not his or her comprehension of a story read aloud, assuming adequate intellectual ability. The decoding problem may be due to a lack of educational exposure, poor educational environment, lack of motivation, and other causes that result in general RD. For example, sociocultural differences

TABLE 1.2   Vision Problems Causing General Reading Dysfunction

Refractive errors (e.g., uncorrected high hyperopia)
Binocular anomalies (e.g., significant convergence insufficiency)
Poor fixations and eye movements (e.g., saccadic undershoots and regressions)
Ocular disease (e.g., cataracts)
Visual perception dysfunctions (e.g., poor visual sequential memory)
Visual-auditory integration dysfunction (e.g., poor sight-sound matching, as shown on the Birch-Belmont test)

may result in poor coding abilities: An individual educated in a foreign language will have decoding difficulties when learning to read and write in English.

Primary emotional or mental health problems often result in general RD, as well as general learning disabilities. In the past, many teachers attributed RD mainly to emotional problems. This misconception may be explained by the realization that RD, particularly dyslexia, often causes *secondary* emotional problems. The optometrist and other professionals on the team should attempt to determine whether there is a primary or secondary emotional problem.

General RD may be the result of certain vision problems, examples of which are listed in Table 1.2. For example, an individual with uncorrected myopia (e.g., −2.00 diopters) may have little problem reading at near distances but would likely have difficulty reading something far away. Astigmatism and hyperopia are likely to contribute to discomfort and inefficiency during the act of reading; the individual generally avoids reading or reads with relatively great difficulty when required to do so. Such refractive errors are likely to result in a general RD. It is our opinion that hyperopia combined with astigmatism may have an even greater deleterious effect than hyperopia alone.

Auditory problems (see Chapter 8) can also result in RD. If auditory acuity is poor, for example, then auditory discrimination of words is poor, which can adversely affect phonologic development in the young child and result in general RD. Auditory problems can also be a factor in dyslexia, particularly in the dysphonetic type of dyslexia. (For discussions of dyslexia, see Chapters 2, 3, and 10.) Poor auditory-visual integrative skills may also result in either general or specific RD.

Attentional and other problems may result in general RD. An attention-deficit disorder (ADD) may or may not have a hyperactivity component. Considerations for ADD in cases of RD are discussed in Chapter 12, in the section on Referral for Educational Therapy.

Because optometrists diagnose and treat vision problems, these causes of general RD are discussed in detail in this book. However,

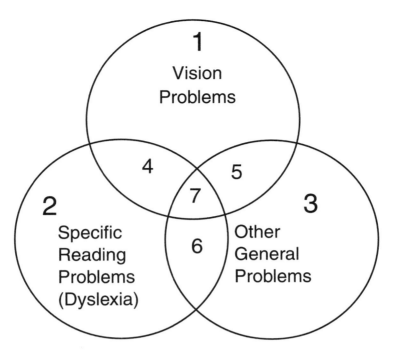

FIGURE 1.1   *Diagram illustrating causes of reading dysfunction.*

other causes of general RD are covered only in a cursory fashion. Optometrists should consider referring patients with general RD to appropriate professionals for treatment of causes such as primary emotional problems, auditory problems, ADD, and allergies. Dyslexia is discussed at length in terms of clinical management and comanagement with other professionals.

Our model is composed of three areas: (1) certain vision problems causing general RD; (2) coding problems of dyslexia causing specific RD; and (3) other problems that cause general RD. This model is depicted in the Venn diagram (Figure 1.1), in which each area of RD is represented within a circle. Position of the circles relative to one another is arbitrary, however optometrists generally explore vision problems before dyslexia or other causes of general RD. An individual's general RD due mainly to vision problems, such as high, uncorrected hyperopic astigmatism and poor visual form discrimination would fall into circle 1. Overlapping areas are represented by numbers 4 through 7. Table 1.3 lists examples of problems that correspond to areas 1–7 in Figure 1.1. Factors within circles 1 or 3 result in general RD. For example, a child who is nondyslexic and has no vision problem but has a severe allergy may have a general problem when reading for any prolonged duration. Similarly, high uncorrected hyperopia could be the cause of a general RD. The optometrist, therefore, should

TABLE 1.3   Examples of Problems Causing Reading Dysfunction (see Figure 1.1)

Segment	Description
1	Vision problems (e.g., convergence insufficiency)
2	Dyslexia (e.g., poor phonetic decoding and encoding)
3	Other problems (e.g., allergies)
4	Vision problems and dyslexia (e.g., convergence insufficiency and dyslexia)
5	Vision and other problems (e.g., convergence insufficiency and allergies)
6	Dyslexia and other problems (e.g., dyslexia and allergies)
7	Vision problems, dyslexia, and other problems (e.g., convergence insufficiency, dyslexia, and allergies)

look for all factors that may be included in circles 1, 2, or 3, and see that they are either ruled in or out.

Summary

Factors listed in Table 1.1 usually cause general RD. Dyslexia is a subtype of RD and is synonymous with specific RD. General RD may be caused by vision problems or other problems. A combination of general and specific RD may exist (for example, a dyslexic individual may also have convergence insufficiency). Optometrists should manage vision-related RD and comanage dyslexic patients with specific RD and patients with general RD due to other problems.

References

1. The 1986/87 Future of Visual Development/Performance Task Force. Special report: the efficacy of optometric vision therapy. J Am Optom Assoc 1988;59:95–105.
2. Bartlett JD. Optometry and literacy (editorial). J Am Optom Assoc 1990;61:82.
3. Grisham JD, Simons HD. Refractive error and the reading process: a literature analysis. J Am Optom Assoc 1986;57:44–55.
4. Simons HD, Grisham JD. Binocular anomalies and reading problems. J Am Optom Assoc 1987;58:578–87.
5. Simons HD, Gassler PA. Vision anomalies and reading skill: a meta-analysis of the literature. Am J Optom Physiol Opt 1988;65:893–904.
6. Harris AJ. How many kinds of reading disability are there? J Learn Disabil 1982;15:456–60.
7. Christenson GN, Griffin JR, Wesson MD. Optometry's role in reading disabilities: resolving the controversy. J Am Optom Assoc 1990;61:363–72.
8. Boder E. Developmental dyslexia: a new diagnostic approach based on the identification of three subtypes. J Sch Health 1970;40:289–90.

9. Griffin JR. Office testing for dyslexia. Curr Opin Ophthalmol 1992;3:111–6.
10. Boder E, Jarrico S. The Boder Test of Reading-Spelling Patterns. New York: Grune & Stratton, 1982.
11. Christenson GN, Griffin JR, De Land PN. Validity of The Dyslexia Screener (TDS). Optom Vis Sci 1991;68:275–81.
12. Guerin DW, Griffin JR, Gottfried AW, et al. Dyslexic subtypes and severity levels: are there gender differences? Optom Vis Sci 1993;70:348–51.
13. Cardinal DN, Christenson GN, Griffin JR. Neurological-behavioral model of dyslexia. J Behav Optom 1992;3:35–9.
14. Griffin JR, Walton HN. The Dyslexia Determination Test (DDT) (rev ed). Los Angeles: Instructional Materials and Equipment Distributors, 1987.
15. Perspectives. Bull Orton Dyslexia Soc 1995;21:3.

2   Literacy Development

Literacy refers to the possession of reading and writing skills adequate to function in educational, vocational, and avocational pursuits. The problem of functional illiteracy (reading below the sixth-grade level) is not limited to underdeveloped nations: An estimated one-fifth to one-third of U.S. citizens are functionally illiterate.[1] Although the lack of written linguistic proficiency is common throughout the world, most people are proficient in the spoken language. Aspects of language acquisition are discussed in this chapter: listening, speaking, reading, and writing. Decoding and comprehension are discussed as they relate to the reading process.

Purpose of Language

Language is necessary for interpersonal communication and individual thinking processes. Chomsky proposed that the nature of language contributes to development of the mind.[2] Acquisition of higher levels of linguistic communication is an arduous task. Many people have great difficulty in achieving higher levels, and some are unable to attain the highest level, linguistic proficiency.

TABLE 2.1   Developmental Stages of Linguistic Skills

Skill Sequence	Normal Onset
Listening (oral receptive)	At birth
Speaking (oral expressive)	Age 1–2 years
Reading (written receptive)	Age 5–6 years
Writing (written expressive)	Age 6–7 years

Development of linguistic skills is categorized into four sequential stages: (1) receptive oral (listening), (2) expressive oral (speaking), (3) receptive written (reading), and (4) expressive written (writing).[2] Individual linguistic development progresses from listening to speaking to reading to writing (Table 2.1).

Spoken Language

An infant begins learning the first stage of communication by hearing nurturing words from a parent, such as *eat, drink,* and *good.* Before the age of 1, the baby learns to babble, and between 12 and 15 months, speaks his or her first words. By the age of 2, a child is usually speaking in fairly complete sentences.[3] Receptive language at this stage is far more advanced than expressive language; for example, a 2-year-old who is shown an apple and asked to name it may have difficulty verbalizing. If the child is asked merely to point to an apple in a basket of various fruits and vegetables, a successful response is much more likely. Even in later life, listening vocabulary exceeds speaking vocabulary. This does not imply that listening is of less value than speaking; in fact, it is necessary for gathering information.

In all probability, speech has been around as long as modern humans have inhabited the earth. Definitive fossil evidence of bone structure necessary for vocalization suggests that Neanderthals may have been speaking 60,000 years ago.[4] There is no group of normal humans who are void of spoken language. All spoken languages are equally complex,[5] and the communication of feelings, desires, requests, commands, and so forth are equally intricate.

Written Language

Compared with speaking, writing is a relatively recent acquisition. Early evidence of written language include pictographic representations, the hieroglyphics of the Egyptians, from about 6000 B.C.

Language	Sentence with Phonetic English
English	The night is beautiful. (thuh nīt iz bū' tuh-fuhl)
Spanish	La noche es hermosa. (lah nō'chĕ ĕs ĕr-mō'sah)
French	La nuit est belle. (lah nū-ĕ' ā bel)
Korean	밤 이 아 름 답 습 니 다 . (bahm ĕ ah rüm dahp süm nĕ dah)
Chinese	今 日 兔 彳民 美 麗 . (chĕng wah ahn mā lĕ) [spoken with variable pitch]
Arabic	هذه ليلة جميلة (hah' thee-hee lay'lah jah-mee' lah)

FIGURE 2.1 *Examples of writing in several languages.*

Gradually, phonetic representations (grapheme-phoneme matches) were written, until alphabets with a limited number of symbols evolved. The oldest written language related to English that has been extensively documented is Sanskrit (about 1500 B.C.). Sanskrit was used in Northern India.[5]

In English, the 26 letters of the alphabet can be used to describe most things in the world. This is highly efficient compared to the approximately 5,000 basic written characters in the Chinese language. The phonetic symbols for a limited alphabet were as significant an advance in literacy as was the introduction of the Arabic decimal system of 10 numbers, which allowed mathematics to flourish.

Most of those formerly pictographic (or logographic) languages have converted to phonetic alphabets (e.g., Korean, the Japanese Kana, and several other Asian languages). Figure 2.1 illustrates the Roman alphabetic system for English, Spanish, and French. These are phonetic lan-

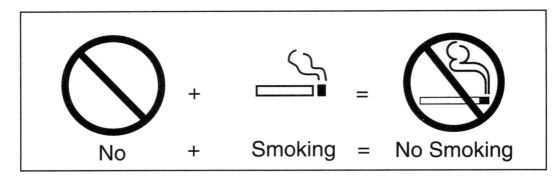

FIGURE 2.2   *Using nonphonetic symbols to convey a message.*

guages, but all have phonetic spelling irregularities, such as the schwa sound for *i* and *u* in beautiful, the silent *h* in hermosa, and the long *a* for *est*. Of these three languages, Spanish is the most phonetically regular, followed by English and French. Korean (see Figure 2.1) uses a different coding system than the Roman alphabet, but it is very regular phonetically (particularly because a strict set of rules is followed in North Korea). Arabic also generally follows regular phonetic rules.

Chinese (see Figure 2.1) is the principal example of a nonphonetic logographic language. The symbols in Figure 2.2 show how universal such logographic languages can be. A nonphonetic logographic written language, such as Chinese, has some advantage over phonetically written ones: The reader does not need to know how to speak the language. The Chinese nation has been held together by its written language when the various spoken dialects would have prevented unification because they are incomprehensible from one region to another. An example of a pictographic sentence is shown in Figure 2.3.[6]

Humans as a species first developed listening and speaking skills, followed by the evolution of reading and writing. Similarly, each individual goes through the same sequence. The duration of each stage may vary from person to person, but the sequence remains the same. Normally, a child begins to decode words and read simple sentences at about the age of 5 or 6. Without acquisition of a spoken language before this stage, it is highly improbable that a child could learn to read. An exception is occasionally found in congenitally deaf individuals whose speech is imperfect. For these individuals, successful reading instruction must include special educational training programs. (Another exception is writing in Chinese or other nonphonetic logographic written languages.)

Spoken English is believed to be more than 1,500 years old, but written English did not come about until a few hundred years later[7] (Table 2.2). Written expression does not occur without reading, but preliterate writing of letters and copying of simple words facilitate the

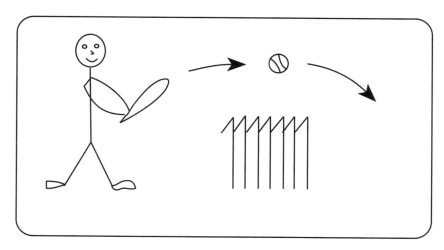

FIGURE 2.3   *The person hits the baseball over the fence. (Reproduced from E Forrest, reported by H Hendrickson. Eponyms of Behavioral Optometry. Santa Ana, CA: Optometric Extension Program Foundation, 1993;27.)*

TABLE 2.2   Evolution of the English Alphabet, Writing, and Spelling

1. Prior to the fourteenth century B.C., the ancient Mongols, Tibetans, or Indians formed the idea of an alphabet instead of logograms (e.g., Egyptian hieroglyphs, Mayan glyphs, Sumerian cuneiforms, and Chinese characters). Logographic examples in modern English include +, –, $, %.

2. 14th century B.C. Syrian coastal town of Ugarit. Cuneiform writing on clay tablets led to Semitic alphabets that used only consonants; dots and lines above or below the consonants indicated vowel sounds. This evolutionary line led to modern Arabic and Hebrew writing systems.

3. 8th century B.C. Greeks were the first to use the same type of letters for all five vowels as those used for consonants.

4. Circa 600 A.D. The evolution from Greek to Roman language eventually led to the first writing system for English speakers. Early missionaries adapted the Roman (Latin) alphabet to Old English; this written language was phonetically regular.

5. 1066, Norman Conquest. From this time on, about half of the English words were borrowed from the French, using French spellings with different rules from those in English. Thus, many modern English words have phonetically irregular spelling.

6. 1755, Samuel Johnson's dictionary. English spelling was standardized; however, pronunciations have changed over time, thus making modern English even more phonetically irregular. (In the German language, spelling changes have evolved with pronunciation changes to keep spelling phonetically regular.)

7. Present. Modern English has become a practical and almost universal language in business, science, aviation, and other areas. It is also a beautiful and eloquent language, but its inconsistent spelling often makes decoding and encoding difficult, especially for dyslexic individuals.

Source: Abstracted and modified from J Diamond. Writing right. Discover 1994;15:106–13.

learning-to-read process. Copying letters requires good visual-motor integration skills (see Chapter 9) so that the physical act of putting pen to paper can be carried out. In the majority of instances, writing is a more challenging task than reading. It is much easier, for example, to read a novel than to write one. Also, a person's reading vocabulary exceeds his or her written vocabulary (especially for correct spelling).

All four stages (listening, speaking, reading, and writing) are necessary for success in a highly literate society. Each successive stage builds on the previous stages. Conversely, the stages of reading and writing help make an individual a better listener and speaker through understanding of syntax, semantics, and acquisition of general and specific information. A case can be made for writing as key to the development of good speaking skills, primarily because there exists a dual system of communication between the spoken and written forms of language. Many more colloquial and nonverbal forms of communication are available in spoken than in written communication. Writing is a necessarily more proper and precise form of expressive communication than is speaking. New ideas and important issues tend to be clarified when they are written down. Thus, speaking becomes more eloquent as a result of writing.

This text is concerned with problems with the *written* language (reading and writing). An overview of the steps in the process of reading follows.

Steps in the Reading Process

According to Tinker,[8] learning to read is a complex developmental process that follows certain stages: (1) the child acquires decoding skills in word recognition; (2) the decoding vocabulary is increased; (3) knowledge of concepts and comprehension of ideas emerge; (4) the older child increases the capacity to grasp meaning and appreciate the style of written passages; and (5) beyond the seventh grade, a mature reader should be able to interpret, evaluate, and reflect on the meaning of what was read. Reading involves two principal processes: *decoding* and *comprehension.* In early grades, reading is heavily dependent on decoding ("bottom-up" processing); in higher grades, comprehension ("top-down" processing) becomes increasingly important[9] (Figure 2.4). We believe the decoding aspects of reading can be included in the optometric realm but that the comprehension aspects belong principally, although not exclusively, in the educational realm. In reading-to-learn tasks, good visual and perceptual-motor skills undoubtedly affect comprehension. Training of these visually related reading skills is in the optometric realm.

Optometrists should keep in mind these five steps in the development of reading. Step 1, decoding, especially concerns the optometrist in clinical practice. (Some aspects of step 1 are listed in Table 2.3.)

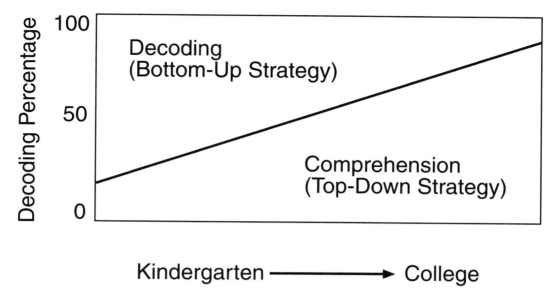

FIGURE 2.4 *Relative importance in reading of decoding (bottom-up strategy) and compre-hension (top-down strategy, such as contextual analysis and the reader's previous knowl-edge of the subject being read). We believe decoding in this paradigm includes both phonetic (syllabic) and eidetic (whole-word) decoding. (Modified from HD Simons. The reading process and learning to read. J Am Optom Assoc 1987;58:883.)*

TABLE 2.3   Areas of Optometric Involvement Relating to Word Recognition in the Reading Process

Visual acuity and lens applications
Peripheral awareness
Eye position maintenance
Eye movements
Accommodation
Vergences
Visual perception (e.g., form discrimination, figure-ground perception)
Visual-motor integration
Auditory-visual integration
Visual-linguistic-cognitive coding of written words (dyslexia testing)

Educators are particularly concerned with the remaining steps. The developmental process of steps 2–5 are thwarted, however, when step 1 has not been developed normally.

Cattell[10] concluded that good readers perceive words as whole units and recognize single words as quickly as single letters. Erdmann and Dodge[11] concurred, finding that subjects could recognize words that were printed in such small type that individual letters could not be identified. Furthermore, a word could be viewed extrafoveally and be recognized, whereas the individual letters could not be. Huey[12] emphasized that a familiar word should be recognized and named just like a familiar object in one's environment. Woodworth and Schlosberg[13] pointed out that both the external configuration of a printed word and its internal patterns must be taken into account. The external outlines of the words *consonants* and *communists* are similar, but the internal patterns are sufficiently different to avoid confusion. Some dyslexics often rely on the template or outline of a word as the role identifer for that word, ignoring the internal patterns.

What part of the word is the most important feature for initial recognition? The root is usually the first syllable in many short words of Old English derivation (e.g., *whaling, toothless*), but words of Latin derivation frequently have the root in the middle, with a prefix before and a suffix after (e.g., *unsuccessful, subservient*). According to Vernon,[14] the most important part depends on the particular word.

Tinker[8] explained the difference between familiar words (referred to by Tinker as sight words) and those that are insufficiently familiar, and hence require phonetic analysis. "The procedure for perception in reading, in which the external outline of the word shape has an important cue value, *operates only for sight words*, those words which have become thoroughly familiar to the reader from meeting them often in his reading." According to Tinker, a child begins to read and continues to add to the bank of sight words throughout his or her lifetime. We refer to this method of word recognition as *eidetic decoding*. Tinker described the situation in which unfamiliar words are encountered:

> *Analysis of them requires rather complete visual scrutiny of the word elements to sound out the word mentally or perhaps subvocally. Having identified the pronunciation, the reader, through use of the verbal context in which the word appears and association with whatever past experience he has had with the sound of the word, achieves meaning and perception.*

This method of word recognition (with some modifications, to be clarified later in this text) is referred to as *phonetic decoding*. There are, therefore, two principal types of linguistic-cognitive decoding: eidetic and phonetic.[15, 16] Decoding is necessary for bottom-up reading, especially in the early school years before comprehension can be used for top-down reading.[16]

Summary

The acquisition of reading and writing—for which listening and speaking are prerequisites—depends on the sequence for the development of linguistic skills. The individual development of linguistic skills recapitulates the development of language in humankind generally. This explains the disparity in difficulty between the attainment of reading and writing skills and the attainment of listening and speaking skills. The process of reading involves several steps. The initial step, word recognition, is the most important for the optometrist to evaluate. Many visual factors affect linguistic processing in this stage. Eidetic and phonetic decoding of words are the two basic visual-linguistic-cognitive processes in word recognition.

References

1. California Literacy Campaign. Bulletin. Placentia, CA: Placentia Library District, 1989.
2. Smith N, Wilson D. Modern Linguistics: Results of Chomsky's Revolution. Bloomington: Indiana University Press, 1980;9.
3. White BL. The First Three Years of Life. Englewood Cliffs, NJ: Prentice-Hall, 1975;173.
4. Geographica. Did Neandertals speak? New bone of contention. National Geographic October, 1989;(suppl):176.
5. Williams JM. Origins of the English Language: A Social and Linguistic History. New York: The Free Press, 1975;46.
6. Hendrickson H. Eponyms of Behavioral Optometry. Santa Ana, CA: Optometric Extension Program Foundation, 1993;27.
7. Diamond J. Writing right. Discover 1994;15:106–13.
8. Tinker MA. Bases for Effective Reading. Minneapolis: University of Minnesota Press, 1965;3–4.
9. Simons HD. The reading process and learning to read. J Am Optom Assoc 1987;58:883–87.
10. Cattell JM. Ueber die Zeit der Erkennung und Benennung won Schriftzeichen, Bildern and Farben. Phil Stud 1885;2:634–50. Cited by MA Tinker. Bases for Effective Reading. Minneapolis: University of Minnesota Press, 1965;15.
11. Erdmann B, Dodge R. Psychologische Untersuchungen ueber das Lesen auf Experimenteller Grundlage. Halle, Belgium: Max Niemeyer, 1898.
12. Huey EB. The Psychology and Pedagogy of Reading, with a Review of the History of Reading and Writing, Texts, and Hygiene in Reading. New York: Macmillan, 1908;75.
13. Woodworth RS, Schlosberg H. Experimental Psychology (rev ed). New York: Holt, Rinehart & Winston, 1954;101.
14. Vernon MD. The Experimental Study of Reading. Cambridge: Cambridge University Press, 1931.
15. Boder E. Developmental Dyslexia: A Diagnostic Screening Procedure Based on Three Characteristic Patterns of Reading and Spelling. In B Bateman (ed), Learning Disorders. Vol 4. Seattle: Special Child Publications, 1971;297–342.
16. Griffin JR, Walton HN. The Dyslexia Determination Test (DDT). Los Angeles: Instructional Materials and Equipment Distributors, 1981 (rev ed, 1987).

3   Theories of Dyslexia

Optometrists examine many patients with reading problems. The terms *specific learning disability*, *reading disability*, and *dyslexia* are included in the Association of Schools and Colleges of Optometry curriculum model for oculomotor, binocular, and visual perceptual dysfunctions.[1] The term *dyslexia* has had almost as many different meanings as there are practitioners. A review in this chapter illustrates the evolution of theoretic knowledge of dyslexia. The discussion in this chapter clarifies an operational definition based on neurologic and behavioral principles. Once dyslexia is defined in clinical terms, the various types of dyslexia can be diagnosed and appropriate management recommendations made. A comparative analysis of the prevalence of types and severity of dyslexia is given.

Visual Factors

Visual disorders such as hyperopia, convergence insufficiency, poor fusional vergence reserves, fixation disparity, hyperphoria, anisometropia, accommodative dysfunctions, poor saccadic eye movements, and inefficient visual perceptual processing, among other dysfunctions, have been shown to adversely affect reading performance and sustainability.[2-11] Obviously, refractive errors, such as hyperopia and astigmatism, can be managed by lens prescriptions. Dysfunctions related to vergence, accommodation, eye movement control, and visual perceptual inefficiencies, however, may be amenable to vision training. An extensive literature review (238 articles) provides evidence that such problems are treatable by means of optometric vision therapy.[12] Nevertheless, some researchers have been neutral or have attempted to discredit the efficacy of optometric vision therapy for the treatment of visual dysfunctions in individuals with learning or reading disabilities.[13-21] In their review of vision therapy, Keogh and Pelland concluded that the role of optometry in the treatment of the learning disabled required clarification.[22] At issue was the need for delineation of which vision therapy procedures are most effective in treating specific vision problems related to learning disabilities.

Optometric vision therapy as a means of reading improvement has been mistakenly associated with controversial regimens involving children who have reading dysfunction (RD).[14, 19] Some of the more controversial treatment modes for dyslexia have included tinted lenses for the "scotopic sensitivity syndrome,"[23] patching an eye to eliminate "unstable ocular dominance,"[24] and eccentric viewing to offset a "foveal neurologic deficit."[25] Other controversial treatments include antivertigo medication to eliminate "inner ear problems,"[26] cross-patterned creeping training for "neurologic organization,"[27] and chiropractic bone manipulation of the skull to release, among other things, an "ocular lock."[28] Rosner and Rosner[23, 29] pointed out the fallacies of these unproved methods for treatment of dyslexia.

Historic Review of Dyslexia

Before the twentieth century, the term *word blindness* was often used in cases of adults who had acquired an inability to read; Berlin introduced the term *dyslexia* in 1887, but it was Hinshelwood who in 1896 differentiated alexia (complete "word blindness") from dyslexia (partial impairment).[30] In 1925, Orton described dyslexia and noted that a person of normal intelligence can have dyslexia.[31] Spache[32] stated that, because of the diversity of meanings and uses of the term *dyslexia*, there was no coherent concept of what it described. Echoing this sentiment, the *Dictionary of Reading and Related Terms*[33] defined dyslexia as follows: "Due to all the differing assumptions about the process and nature of possible reading problems, dyslexia has come to have so many incompatible connotations that it has lost any real value for educators except as a fancy word for a reading problem."

TABLE 3.1   Overview of Theories of Dyslexia

Date	Name	Theory
1925	Orton	Incomplete cerebral dominance
1925–1959	Monroe	Developmental lag
	Fernald	Developmental lag
	Bender	Developmental lag
1960–1969	Barsch	Incomplete perceptual development
	Delacato	Incomplete perceptual development
	Frostig	Incomplete perceptual development
	Getman	Incomplete perceptual development
	Cruickshank	Incomplete perceptual development
	Kirk	Psycholinguistic problems
	Wepman	Auditory discrimination problems
	de Hirsch	Language problems
	Myklebust	Language problems
	Bateman	Language problems
1970–present	Keogh	Attention problems
	Margolis	Attention problems
	Bannatyne	Poor memory
	Vellutino	Language disorders
	Satz	Maturational lag
	Torgesen	Mismatch in abilities and education

Source: Modified from K Koenke. Dyslexia: a view of the theories. J Reading 1983;27:274–7.

The lack of a coherent concept of dyslexia in the past is further illustrated by viewing the various theories of its etiology, prepared by Koenke,[34] in Table 3.1. Adelman and Taylor[35] and Kolb and Whishaw[36] underscored the basis for this confusion by stating that most people use *dyslexia* as a label for everyone who has a reading problem rather than reserving it for individuals who have a specific central nervous system (CNS) dysfunction.

Efforts have been made to segregate nondyslexic poor readers from dyslexics (who are necessarily poor readers) in an attempt to clarify the effects of CNS dysfunction as opposed to other causal factors, such as educational deprivation and primary emotional problems. In this vein, Critchley[37] proposed a diagnosis of dyslexia as "a disorder manifested by difficulty in learning to read despite conventional instruction, adequate intelligence, and sociocultural opportunity. It is dependent upon fundamental cognitive abilities which frequently are constitutional in origin." This definition gives rise to two broad categories of RD: nonspecific RD and specific RD (dyslexia). The nonspecific types are reading problems that result from one or more of the etiologies listed in Critchley's definition: lack of educational opportunity, low intelligence, and sociocultural deprivation (see Chapter 1). We include attentional and vision problems in this list as possible causes of nonspecific RD.

Attentional deficits can cause general RD. They also cause general learning disabilities.[38] Effects of attentional deficits are discussed in Chapter 12.

Dyslexia may be characterized as a specific RD, but it can further be defined as a deficit in an individual's ability to interpret the symbols of written language due to minimal brain dysfunction or differential brain function.[39] Differential brain function implies that an individual may be good at some activities and poor at others, as in music versus math. Accordingly, a dyslexic individual displays a characteristic pattern of decoding (recognizing) and encoding (spelling) difficulties with written words. Types of coding patterns are discussed in the next section of this chapter.

There are three general methods for diagnosis of dyslexia: (1) exclusionary diagnosis, (2) indirect diagnosis, and (3) direct diagnosis. In the exclusionary diagnosis, all the factors involved in nonspecific RD (vision and other general contributory problems) must be ruled out to make the diagnosis of dyslexia. The exclusionary method is one step in the diagnosis, but it neither provides a direct diagnosis nor identifies the type of dyslexia. A more specific method of diagnosing the dyslexic population is also needed. Indirect approaches, such as finger agnosia (identification of a nonviewed finger when it is touched), attempted to associate such neurologic "soft" signs with reading failure.[40] Such indirect approaches have been unsuccessful because many dyslexics do not manifest such neurologic signs. Other unsuccessful indirect approaches have used cluster analysis of cognitive testing, such as comparing subtests within the intelligence tests to identify specific characteristics of dyslexia.[41, 42] Attempts to relate overall IQ to reading achievement and potential have not been fruitful for dyslexics.[43]

The most reliable and efficacious diagnostic method for dyslexia is the direct method. This approach involves the use of characteristic decoding and encoding patterns that directly determine the specific dyslexic type.[39, 43–51] The direct diagnostic method reveals that dyslexia is a heterogeneous, rather than homogeneous, disorder. Each of the several types of dyslexia has its own distinct pattern of reading and spelling failure.[39, 44–51]

Neurologic-Behavioral Model

Types of dyslexia are based on validation of two distinct cognitive processes for decoding and encoding of words: (1) phonologic (*phonetic*) and (2) orthographic or whole-word (*eidetic*).[39, 44–54] There is a neurophysiologic and anatomic basis for these two linguistic-cognitive coding functions.[46, 47, 51–57] Much of the phonetic coding function is harbored in Wernicke's area of the left temporal lobe; much of the eidetic coding function is mediated by the angular gyrus of the left parietal lobe.[39, 47, 52–54]

TABLE 3.2   Some Proponents of Types of Dyslexia

Proponents	Types
Camp and Dolcourt[49] (1977)	Eidetic and phonetic
Boder[45] (1982)	Eidetic and phonetic
Hynd and Hynd[46] (1984)	Surface and phonologic (deep)
Roeltgen and Heilman[47] (1984)	Lexical and phonologic
Temple[50] (1984)	Surface and phonologic
Griffin and Walton[39] (1981)	Eidetic and phonetic
Flynn and Deering[51] (1989)	Eidetic and phonetic

Boder[44, 45] reported this model of phonetic and eidetic processing of words in the early 1970s. Caution was advised, however, in accepting the validity of this classification scheme.[58] Many authorities nevertheless have come to agree with this classification model, inconsistencies of labeling notwithstanding. Table 3.2 lists some of the proponents of the eidetic and phonetic classification schemes of word coding.[39, 44, 46–51] Although terminology may differ among these proponents, the basis for classification is similar.

The two decoding functions, eidetic and phonetic, are integrally involved in the bottom-up process of reading. Top-down processing theoretically involves comprehension (rather than decoding)—that is, the use of contextual analysis, semantics, and syntax. Obviously, if a significant number of words are not decoded, the individual will have comprehension problems.

Since the late 1980s, the top-down process has been emphasized in education, often at the expense of teaching children the bottom-up process. This top-down process is known as the literature-based "whole-language" approach. According to Simons, "there is still substantial support in the reading literature for the importance of bottom-up processing and decoding instruction."[59] Simons further stated, "Optometrists visiting learning disability classes, reading clinics, and talking to reading specialists in the schools will find that the inability to decode is the problem most often cited for the reading problems of many children." The recent trend of the literature-based whole-language approach in education may further exacerbate the problem of poor decoding skills, particularly for dyslexics, because the approach does not emphasize these skills.

A knowledge of brain function in reading is important to understanding the specific difficulties experienced by people with dyslexia. Hynd and Hynd pointed out the need for greater awareness: "Much if not all of the recent research conducted by neuroscientists is ignored in favor of a simplistic view of dyslexia."[46]

For general understanding of the types of dyslexia, it is helpful to review the theory of basic brain function. There have been two schools of thought. The first is the localizationist theory espoused by Gall,[60] although his phrenologic concept is no longer accepted. Broca,[61] Wernicke,[62] and Jackson,[63] among others, investigated localized areas of the brain, rather than the skull. Their basic tenet was that the brain is compartmentalized and that specific behavioral and cognitive functions are represented in discrete brain locations. Supporting this theory is the fact that damage to specific brain areas causes predictable behavioral changes. This theory remained in scientific favor until the advent of the post–World War I Gestalt movement. Lashley's theory of "mass action"[64] evolved during this time. Lashley's fundamental premise was that the site of a brain lesion is unimportant; rather, the mass of brain tissue involved is the critical factor in determining which behavioral deficits ensue.

Heilman and Valenstein[65] reported a reawakening of the localizationist theory based on the following: (1) replicable behavioral changes associated with circumscribed brain lesions, (2) technologic advances allowing for improved scientific study of brain-behavior relationships (e.g., computed tomography scans and electroencephalographic techniques), and (3) pathologic and cytoarchitectonic studies of the brain.

The consensus theory includes both the mass actionists and the localizationists, as summarized by Luria:[66] "The material basis of the higher nervous processes is the brain as a whole but the brain is a highly differentiated system whose parts are responsible for the action of the whole." This theory is applicable to the coding processes involved in reading, writing, and spelling.

Types of Dyslexia

Research has demonstrated specific cortical locations, principally in the left hemisphere of the brain (for right-handed and most left-handed individuals), that appear to be primarily responsible for the two fundamental linguistic-cognitive processes. These processes have been described as (1) phonetic (syllabic) word analysis and (2) eidetic (whole-word) analysis. The dynamics of these two processes become evident in the explanation of how words are decoded based on the neurologic-behavioral model of Griffin and Walton.[39] A visual configuration of a word, represented by a grouping of letters, is processed through the primary visual pathway and associated areas. Impulses are then transmitted to the angular gyrus of the left parietal lobe, where a sight-sound match may be made if the word is one with which the patient is sufficiently familiar. If such a match is made (within 1–2 seconds) the word is said to have been in the individual's sight-word vocabulary and is processed eidetically. For unfamiliar words, more extensive analysis is required; Wernicke's area mediates the phonetic analysis (word attack). This generally requires more than

TABLE 3.3   Basic Types of Dyslexia

Type	Anatomic Location	Affected Coding Process
Dyseidesia	Angular gyrus of left parietal lobe (for right handers)	Eidetic (whole word)
Dysphonesia	Wernicke's area of left temporal and parietal lobes (for right handers)	Phonetic (syllabic)
Dysnemkinesia	Motor cortex of frontal lobe (left hemisphere) for right handers	Motoric memory of letter formations

Source: JR Griffin, HN Walton. The Dyslexia Determination Test (DDT) (rev ed). Los Angeles: Instructional Materials and Equipment Distributors, 1987.

1–2 seconds because the word must be syllabicated—that is, each syllable is sounded out and then the sounds for each syllable are blended. Note that there are irregular English words that are difficult to attack phonetically, such as the word *should* (which sounds as though it were written as "shud").

A third area of linguistic processing occurs in the motor cortex, which is assumed to be where motor engrams for the duplication of letter forms are developed, stored, and called on when writing words.[39] Letter reversals during writing may be attributed, in part, to inadequate development of these motor engrams. A dyslexia of this type is called *dysnemkinesia* (literally meaning poor memory of movement). Many individuals with dyslexia do not exhibit these reversal problems to an abnormal degree. (See Table 3.3 for a synopsis of the types of dyslexia and the neuroanatomic substrate and coding process affected for each type.)

Based on the neuroanatomic model described, three basic types of dyslexia may be identified by direct diagnostic testing. One type is called *dyseidesia*,[39, 44, 45, 49, 51] and is related to minimal brain dysfunctions or differential brain function that appear to be in the angular gyrus. The characteristic reading, writing, and spelling problems deficits associated with dyseidesia are based on the functions subserved by the above-mentioned cortical area. For example, an individual with a dysfunction in the angular gyrus of the left parietal lobe has difficulty processing words eidetically (making an immediate sight-sound match). Such an affected individual has poor sight-word recognition and relies on time-consuming word-attack skills (phonetic approach) to decode many words. The result is laborious reading, which understandably diminishes comprehension. Decoding becomes inaccurate for many phonetically irregular words (e.g., *log* for *laugh*). Such individuals are poor in look-say decoding. Characteristic spelling errors include the reliance on phonetic equivalents for irregular words (e.g., *rede* for *ready)* (Figure 3.1).

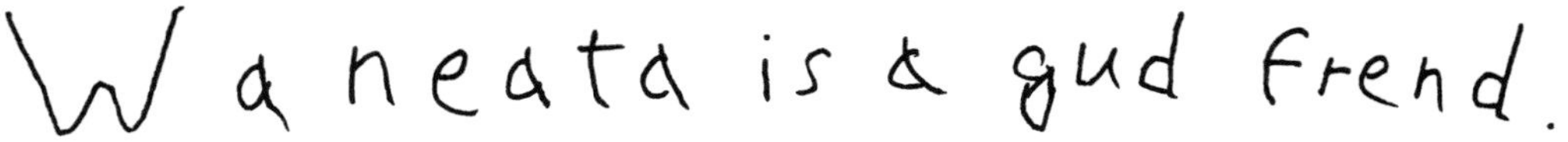

Waneata is a gud frend.

FIGURE 3.1 *Typical spelling errors in dyseidesia. (Assume student is in the fourth grade in Figures 3.12 through 3.7.) Note that good phonetic equivalents were achieved, but there are problems with eidetic revisualization. The patient was attempting to write, "Juanita is a good friend." Although this writing would possibly be expected in a first- or second-grade student, it is not appropriate for a fourth-grade student.*

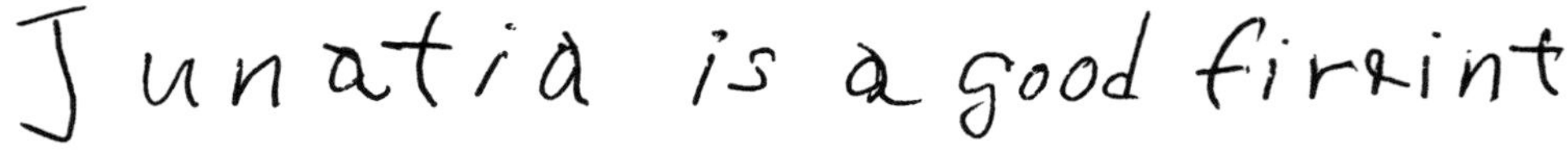

Junatia is a good firxint

FIGURE 3.2 *Typical spelling errors in dysphonesia. Note that there are problems in writing good phonetic equivalents, but attempts were made for eidetic recall (i.e., letters revisualized but transposed).*

A dysfunction in Wernicke's area of the left temporal and parietal lobes is called *dysphonesia*. Individuals with this type of dyslexia have an impairment in phonetic ability to decode unfamiliar words, although eidetic processing (look-say) is intact. [39, 44, 45, 49, 51, 53, 54] The dysphonetic individual characteristically either knows a word as a part of his or her sight-word lexicon or does not. When presented with an unfamiliar written word, even if it is a phonetically regular word (e.g., stop, did, going), a dysphonetic individual may have great difficulty syllabicating, sounding out, and blending the sounds together to decode the word. Typical reading errors are semantic substitutions (e.g., *home* for *house)* due to dependency on contextual clues (i.e., top-down strategy in reading) when undecoded words require guessing. Characteristic spelling errors (Figure 3.2) include nonphonetic equivalents (e.g., *solw* for *slow*). Letter transposition is a common encoding error in dysphonesia.

Dysnemkinesia is presumably due principally to a dysfunction in the portion of the motor cortex involving letter formation.[39] Dysnemkinesia is characterized by an abnormally high frequency of letter reversals (Figure 3.3), (e.g., *d* for *b*, as in writing *doy* for *boy*).

Additional types of dyslexia result from minimal brain dysfunction or differential brain function, or both, occurring in more than one of the three dysfunctioning brain areas to cause a combination of coding errors. *Dysphoneidesia, dysnemkineidesia, dysnemkinphonesia,* and *dysnemkinphoneidesia* are characteristic combinations of the three basic dyslexic types. Permutations of the three basic types, therefore,

Tuanita iz a Goob 7RienD.

FIGURE 3.3 *Example of typical reversal errors in dysnemkinesia. Note that spelling is correct, but there are some letter reversals.*

Wnata is a god fnd.

FIGURE 3.4 *Typical spelling errors in a mixed type of dyslexia called dysphoneidesia. Note that there are problems both in writing revisualized words orthographically and producing good phonetic equivalents.*

Waneata iz a quD 7ReND

FIGURE 3.5 *Typical spelling errors in dysnemkineidesia (combination of dysnemkinesia and dyseidesia). Note the misspelled words with good phonetic equivalents as well as letter reversals.*

Tunatia iz a goob 7ireint

FIGURE 3.6 *Typical spelling errors in dysnemkinphonesia (combination of dysnemkinesia and dysphonesia). Note the poor phonetic equivalents but with attempts made for eidetic recall (i.e., letters revisualized but transposed). Letter reversals are also evident.*

give rise to seven types of dyslexia, each having its own characteristic pattern, which can be defined behaviorly (see Figures 3.1 through 3.7).

Further neurophysiologic support for subtyping of dyslexia has been provided by research, including event-related potential waveforms that differentiate dysphonetic from dyseidetic types.[51, 67, 68]

The Dyslexia Determination Test (DDT)[39] and the Boder Test of Reading-Spelling Patterns[45] provide a direct diagnostic profile of the

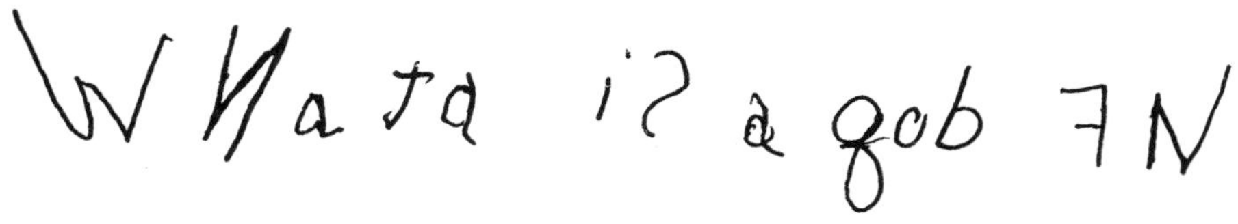

FIGURE 3.7 *Typical spelling errors in dysnemkinphoneidesia (combination of all three basic types, and the most severe type of dyslexia). Note letter reversals, poor phonetic equivalents, and poor eidetic revisualization.*

dyslexic types of dyseidesia and dysphonesia based on the characteristic decoding and encoding patterns manifested during test performance. Testing time for each test is approximately 30 minutes. All types, including dysnemkinesia, can be diagnosed using the DDT. Dysnemkinesia can be determined by evaluating the individual for reversal tendencies in writing letters and numbers.[39] For rapid detection of dyseidesia, dysphonesia, and dysphoneidesia, a screening for these dyslexic types can be performed with high sensitivity and specificity in less than 5 minutes using The Dyslexia Screener (TDS).[69, 70] Note that some authors of this book are coauthors of the DDT or TDS. Their research and clinical testing led to development of these assessment tools.

As discussed previously, factors such as lack of educational opportunity, sensory impairment, and sociocultural deprivation must also be ruled out in all cases of learning and reading disability. With these considerations addressed we have found the diagnosis of specific types of dyslexia consistently repeatable on retesting. This is especially true of dyseidesia, which is reported to be genetically inherited in an autosomal dominant mode of transmission.[71] Dysphonesia and dysnemkinesia are more environmentally influenced than is dyseidesia.[39] Dysnemkinesia is the most strongly environmentally influenced and can usually be modified with therapy directed toward visual-motor and visual-perceptual skills enhancement. Dysphonesia is generally more difficult to resolve than dysnemkinesia and requires a specialized educational approach, as does dyseidesia, the most difficult of the three basic types to resolve (see Chapter 12 for management of dyslexia).

This model of dyslexic subtypes is in accord with current understanding of neurologic processing and behavioral outcomes in reading. There is no other reliable model for the clinical application for direct diagnosis and management of dyslexia.

Prevalence of Dyslexia

Prevalence of any disease or condition can be determined with knowledge of the exact diagnosis and the specified severity level. The

TABLE 3.4   Prevalence of Dyslexia (all types) in Elementary School[39, 70, 72, 73]

Two Regular Third-Grade Classrooms (N = 47)	Prevalence (%)
Borderline or worse severity	23.0
Borderline to mild or worse	12.8
Mild or worse	8.5
Mild to moderate or worse	4.2
Moderate or worse	0.0

Resource Specialist Classroom (N = 21)	
Borderline or worse severity	71.4
Borderline to mild or worse	61.9
Mild or worse	57.1
Mild to moderate or worse	52.4
Moderate or worse	33.3
Moderate to marked or worse	28.6
Marked	9.5

type of dyslexia (e.g., dyseidesia or dysphonesia) and severity (e.g., mild or marked) must be considered. Table 3.4 compares prevalence according to severity (for dysphonetic, dyseidetic, and dysphoneidetic types) in regular and resource (special education) classrooms. Both prevalence and severity were greater in the resource classroom. Although not shown in Table 3.4, severe types of dyslexia (dysphoneidesia being more severe than dyseidesia, and dyseidesia being more severe than dysphonesia) were also more prevalent in the resource classroom.[70, 72–74] Table 3.5 compares prevalence of dyslexia in males in regular high-school classrooms with age-matched juvenile hall (detention center)–incarcerated subjects. Higher prevalence of dyslexia was found in those in the juvenile hall. Although not shown in Table 3.5, there were greater degrees of severity and more severe types of dyslexia in subjects in the juvenile hall.[72, 73] Other studies we have conducted indicate that, when cultural barriers (e.g., bilingualism and lack of education) are accounted for, dyslexia is the main problem in adult literacy programs.[72–74] In school-aged subjects, Guerin et al.[75, 76] found no significant difference in prevalence between genders, but males did have more severe degrees and types of dyslexia than females.

The high prevalence of dyslexia notwithstanding, Swan[77] pointed out that there are probably many more cases of "reading difficulty" than "reading dysfunction" (which he referred to as dyslexia). The implication is that the prevalence of general RD is higher than that of specific RD.

TABLE 3.5   Dyslexia in High School[72, 73]

Males in Regular Midgrouping High-School Classrooms (N = 39)	Prevalence (%)
Borderline or worse severity	18.0
Mild or worse	2.6
Moderate or worse	0.0
Marked or worse	0.0
Males in a Juvenile Hall (N = 40)	
Borderline or worse severity	45.0
Mild or worse	22.5
Moderate or worse	17.5
Marked or worse	7.5

Summary

Dyslexia is not a homogeneous disorder but rather consists of separate, validated types, based on a neurologic-behavioral model. Dyslexia is a separate entity and is not caused by visual dysfunctions, but visual dysfunctions can contribute to the RD of a dyslexic individual, as they do in nondyslexic individuals who have RD due to other factors. In some instances, the main cause of an individual's reading problem may be inefficient visual skills or visual-perceptual-motor dysfunctions. Characteristic coding patterns are evident for the various types of dyslexia. Some types of dyslexia are more genetic in etiology than others. Inherited types of dyslexia are usually more difficult to manage than are the relatively environmental types. Prevalence of dyslexia must be based on severity. Dyslexia is more common in resource rooms than in regular classrooms. There is no gender difference in prevalence, but severity is usually greater in males than in females.

References

1. Flax N, Garzia R, Grisham JD, et al. Curriculum model for oculomotor, binocular, and visual perception dysfunctions. J Optom Educ 1988;13:95–103.
2. Grisham JD, Simons HD. Refractive error and the reading process: a literature analysis. J Am Optom Assoc 1986;57:44–55.
3. Walton HN, Schubert DG. What every teacher should know about hyperopia. Calif Reader 1989;22:20–2.
4. Simons HD, Grisham JD. Binocular anomalies and reading problems. J Am Optom Assoc 1987;58:578–87.

5. Flax N. Visual function in dyslexia. Am J Optom Arch Am Acad Optom l968;45:574–86.
6. Flax N. Problems in relating visual function to reading disorder. Am J Optom Arch Am Acad Optom 1970;47:366–72.
7. Flax N. The eye and learning disabilities. J Am Optom Assoc 1972;43:612–7.
8. Flax N, Mozlin R, Solan HA. Discrediting the basis of the AAO policy. Learning disabilities, dyslexia, and vision. J Am Optom Assoc 1984;55:399–403.
9. Simons HD, Gassler PA. Vision anomalies and reading skill: a meta-analysis of the literature. Am J Optom Physiol Opt l988;65:893–904.
10. Griffin DC, Walton HN, Ives V. Saccades as related to reading disorders. J Learn Disabil 1974;7:310–6.
11. Harris AJ. How many kinds of reading disability are there? J Learn Disabil 1982;15:456–60.
12. Special report: the efficacy of optometric vision therapy, the 1986/87 future of visual development performance task force. J Am Optom Assoc 1988;59:95–105.
13. American Academy of Pediatrics, American Academy of Ophthalmology and Otolaryngology, and American Association of Ophthalmology, joint organization statement on the eye and learning disabilities. Pediatr News 1972;6:63–6.
14. American Academy of Ophthalmology. Policy statement: learning disabilities, dyslexia, and vision. J Learn Disabil 1987;20:412–3.
15. Goldberg HK. Dyslexia and learning disabilities. Pediatr Clin North Am 1983;30:1195–1200.
16. Kavale K, Mattson PD. "One jumped off the balance beam": meta analysis of perceptual-motor training. J Learn Disabil 1983;16:165–73.
17. Helveston EM, Weber JC, Miller K, et al. Visual function and academic performance. Am J Ophthalmol 1985;99:346–55.
18. Helveston EM. Management of dyslexia and related learning disabilities. J Learn Disabil 1987;20:415–21.
19. Silver LB. The "magic cure": a review of the current controversial approaches for treating learning disabilities. J Learn Disabil 1987;20:498–504,512.
20. Vellutino FR. Dyslexia. Sci Am 1987;256:34–41.
21. Casbergue RM, Greene JF. Persistent misconceptions about sensory perception and reading disability. J Reading 1988;32:198–203.
22. Keogh BK, Pelland M. Vision training revisited. J Learn Disabil 1985;18:228–36.
23. Rosner J, Rosner J. The Irlen treatment: a review of the literature. Optician 1987;194:26–33.
24. Stein J, Fowler S. Effect of monocular occlusion on visuomotor perception and reading in dyslexic children. Lancet 1985;13:69–73.
25. Geiger G, Lettvin JY. Peripheral vision in persons with dyslexia. N Engl J Med 1987;316:1238–43.
26. Frank J, Levinson HN. Seasickness mechanisms and medications in dysmetric dyslexia and dyspraxia. Acad Ther 1976;12:133–53.
27. Delacato CH. The Diagnosis and Treatment of Speech and Reading Problems. Springfield, IL: Thomas, 1963.
28. Ferreri CA, Wainwright RD. Breakthrough for Dyslexia and Learning Disabilities. Pompano Beach, FL: Exposition Press of Florida, 1984.

29. Rosner J, Rosner J. Another cure for dyslexia? (editorial). J Am Optom Assoc 1988;59:832–4.
30. Hinshelwood J. A case of dyslexia: a peculiar form of wordblindness. Lancet 1896;2:1451.
31. Orton ST. "Word-blindness" in school children. Arch Neurol Psychiatry 1925;15:581–615.
32. Spache GD. Investigating the Issues of Reading Disabilities. Boston: Allyn & Bacon, 1976.
33. Harris TL, Hodges RE (eds). A Dictionary of Reading and Related Terms. Newark, DE: International Reading Association, 1981.
34. Koenke K. Dyslexia: A view of the theories. J Reading 1983;27:274–7.
35. Adelman HS, Taylor L. The problems of definition and differentiation and the need for a classification schema. J Learn Disabil 1986;19:514–20.
36. Kolb B, Whishaw IQ. Fundamentals of Human Neuropsychology. San Francisco: Freeman, 1980.
37. Critchley M. The Dyslexic Child (2nd ed). Springfield, IL: Thomas, 1970.
38. Steinman BA, Steinman SB, Garzia RP, et al. Vision and reading III: visual attention. J Optom Vision Dev 1996;27:4–28.
39. Griffin JR, Walton HN. The Dyslexia Determination Test (DDT) (rev ed). Los Angeles: Instructional Materials and Equipment Distributors, 1987.
40. Lindgren SD. Finger localization and prediction of reading disability. Cortex 1978;14:87–101.
41. Vance HB, Fuller GB. Discriminant function analysis of LD/ED children scores on WISC-R. J Clin Psychol 1983;39:749–53.
42. Lufli D, Cohen A, Ellis R. Differential diagnosis of learning disability versus emotional disturbance using the WISC-R. J Learn Disabil 1988;21:515–6.
43. Share DL, McGee R, Silva PA. IQ and reading progress: a test of the capacity notion of IQ. J Am Acad Child Adolesc Psychiatry 1989;28:97–100.
44. Boder E. Developmental dyslexia: a diagnostic approach based on three atypical reading patterns. Dev Med Child Neurol 1973;15:663–87.
45. Boder E, Jarrico S. The Boder Test of Reading-Spelling Patterns. New York: Grune & Stratton, 1982.
46. Hynd GW, Hynd CR. Dyslexia: neuroanatomical/neurolinguistic perspectives. Reading Res Q 1984;19:482–98.
47. Roeltgen DP, Heilman KM. Lexical agraphia: further support for the two-system hypothesis of linguistic agraphia. Brain 1984;107:811–27.
48. Johnson DJ, Myklebust HR. Learning Disabilities. New York: Grune & Stratton, 1967;173.
49. Camp BW, Dolcourt JL. Reading and spelling in good and poor readers. J Learn Disabil 1977;10:300–7.
50. Temple CM. New approaches to the developmental dyslexias. Adv Neurol 1984;42:223–32.
51. Flynn JM, Deering WM. Subtypes of dyslexia: investigation of Boder's classification system using quantitative neurophysiology. Dev Med Child Neurol 1989;31:215–23.
52. Geschwind N. Specializations of the human brain. Sci Am 1979;241:180–99.
53. Shallice T. Phonological agraphia and the lexical route in writing. Brain (Oxford) 1981;104:413–29.

54. Roeltgen DP, Sevush S, Heilman KM. Phonological agraphia: writing by the lexical semantic route. Neurology 1983;33:755–65.
55. Duffy FH, Denckla MB, Bartels PH, et al. Dyslexia: automated diagnosis by computerized classification of brain electrical activity. Ann Neurol 1980;7:421–8.
56. Galaburda AM, Kemper TL. Cytoarchitectonic abnormalities in developmental dyslexia: a case study. Ann Neurol 1979;6:94–100.
57. Galaburda AM, Eidelberg D. Symmetry and asymmetry in the human posterior thalamus: II. Thalamic lesions in a case of developmental dyslexia. Arch Neurol 1982;39:333–6.
58. Satz P, Morris R. Learning Disability Subtypes: A Review. In FJ Pirozzolo, MC Wittrock (eds), Neuropsychological and Cognitive Processes in Reading. Orlando, FL: Academic, 1981;109–41.
59. Simons HD. The reading process and learning to read. J Am Optom Assoc 1987;58:883–7.
60. Gall FJ. Sur les fonction du cerveau et sur cells de ses parties. (V. 106). Paris: Bailliere, 1825.
61. Broca P. Nouvelle observation d'amphemine produite par une lesion de la moite posteriure des deuxeme et troisieme circonvolutins frontales. Bull Mem Soc Anat Paris 1861;36:398–407.
62. Wernicke C. Der aphasiche Symptomenkomplex. Breslau, Germany: Cohn & Weigert, 1874.
63. Jackson JH. Case of large cerebral tumor without optic neuritis and without left hemiplegia and imperception. Royal London Ophthalmic Hosp Rep 1876;8:434.
64. Lashley KS. Factors limiting recovery after central nervous lesions. J Nerv Ment Dis 1938;88:733–55.
65. Heilman KM, Valenstein E (eds). Clinical Neuropsychology. New York: Oxford University Press, 1979.
66. Luria AR. Higher Cortical Functions in Man (2nd ed rev). New York: Basic Books, 1980.
67. Fried I, Tanguay PE, Boder E, et al. Development of dyslexia: electrophysiological evidence of clinical subgroups. Brain Lang 1981;12:14–22.
68. Rosenthal JH. EEG Event-Related Potentials in Dyslexia and its Subtypes. In DAB Lindberg, MF Collen, EE Van Brunt (eds), AMIA Congress on Medical Informatics (1st:1982:San Francisco). New York: Masson Pub, 1982.
69. Griffin JR, Walton HN, Christenson GN. The Dyslexia Screener (TDS). Culver City, CA: Reading and Perception Therapy Center, 1988.
70. Christenson GN, Griffin JR, De Land PN. Validity of the dyslexia screener. Optom Vis Sci 1991;68:275–81.
71. Griffin JR. Genetics of dyseidetic dyslexia. Optom Vis Sci 1992;69:148–51.
72. Griffin JR. Prevalence of Dyslexia. Presented at Annual Meeting of the American Public Health Association, Washington, D.C., Nov. 9, 1992.
73. Griffin JR. Prevalence of dyslexia. J Optom Vision Dev 1992;23:17–22.
74. Brin B, Griffin J, Guerin DW. Mass screening for dyslexia. Presented at Annual Meeting of the American Public Health Association, Washington, D.C., Nov. 11, 1992.
75. Guerin DW, Griffin JR, Gottfried AW, et al. Concurrent validity and screening efficiency of the dyslexia screener. Psychol Assessment 1993;5:369–73.

76. Guerin DW, Griffin JR, Gottfried AW, et al. Dyslexic subtypes and severity levels: are there gender differences? Optom Vis Sci 1993;70:348–51.
77. Swan, M. Emergent literacy to reading fluency: climbing the developmental ladder. Ellerbrock Memorial Continuing Education Course #PC-20, Dec. 10, 1994. American Academy of Optometry Meeting, San Diego, CA.

II. Physical and Physiologic Processes in Reading

4 Physical and Physiologic Aspects of Reading

This chapter summarizes some prerequisites of visual information processing related to reading. Although there is evidence for visual processing deficits causing reading dysfunction, some authorities have questioned this role.[1-7]

Mary had a little lamb.   (18 point)

Now is the time for all good people...   (10 point)

FIGURE 4.1   *Eighteen-point primer text compared with 10-point standard text.*

Characteristics of Print as Stimuli to Reading

The physical characteristics of visual stimuli in reading material play an important part in the interpretation of what is read. Type size, print contrast, and quality of paper contribute to readability.

Type Size

Larger sizes of type are usually used for the beginning reader. The larger sizes enhance the decoding process necessary to meaningful comprehension of the text (Figure 4.1).

Although no studies exist to validate this claim, it has been reported that increasing the isolation of printed symbols results in improved visual acuity responses.[8, 9] (This effect is dramatically demonstrated in amblyopia.[10, 11]) It stands to reason that fewer characters on a given line of reading material allow for easier differentiation of letters and syllables. The relatively easy differentiation of letters and syllables, due to the limited number of characters per line, facilitates the grapheme-phoneme matching necessary for decoding. Finishing a page of print gives the new reader a feeling of accomplishment even though there may be fewer than 10 words on that page.

Print Contrast

Size is not the only legibility and efficiency determinant. Another important quality of print is contrast, which may be thought of as the sharpness of type outline against the background of the page. The border of a letter represents a contrast gradient against the background. This is not an absolute knife-edge border, but a nondiscrete edge that can be denoted mathematically.[12, 13] In visual science terms, the edges of letters generate high spatial frequencies, and it is these high spatial frequencies that assist visual resolution of the border of a letter.[14] Within the borders of the printed letter, however, visual resolution relies on middle and low spatial frequencies. The entire spatial fre-

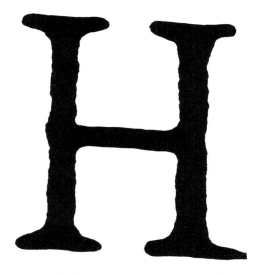

Hospital

FIGURE 4.2 *Enlargement of the letter H from ordinary newspaper print demonstrating loss of edge continuity.*

quency range for a printed letter, therefore, can be analyzed mathematically into discrete components by a Fourier transform.[14] Sharp borders with high spatial frequencies are necessary for efficient reading. For ordinary objects in our environment, however, visual recognition is principally due to midspatial frequencies.[15]

In terms of spatial frequency, 27 cycles per degree (cpd) is approximately 20/20 (6/6) visual acuity. Recognition of most objects in our environment, however, requires only about 6 cpd.[15] This is about one-fourth the spatial frequency resolution optometrists typically expect of patients who perform adequately on a routine vision examination. Therefore, an individual with 20/80 (6/24) corrected acuity should theoretically have adequate sight for many tasks, including reading relatively large newspaper and magazine print. This degree of visual acuity, however, is usually insufficient for most reading tasks. Reading efficiency is affected by degradation of the edges of letters. Even in good quality print, the borders of printed letters are not knife-edged, as can be seen under magnification (Figure 4.2).

Quality of Paper

Characteristics of paper also affect print contrast. The ability of the paper to absorb ink without spreading is desirable. This ensures that the edges of the print remain sharply defined and, thus, maintain high spatial frequency components. Furthermore, glare from the surface of the paper reduces contrast. High-gloss paper creates this problem and can adversely affect reading efficiency.

Light Source

Conventional forms of reading (not including braille) require a source of reflected divergent light on the printed page. That light is mediated by the optical components of the eye and should be properly focused and not degraded by opacities of the ocular media (e.g., cataracts). Transmission of light energy from the printed page to the retina can be thought of as the optical portion of the modulation transfer function (MTF),[14] which is related to visual contrast sensitivity. Even in a properly focusing and opacity-free normal eye, the transfer of light energy to the retinal surface is never 100%. For each energy interface transfer, the MTF modifies the output of the preceding system. Much of the light energy is filtered by the optical system of the eye before reaching the retina. Ametropia and abnormalities of the ocular media further exacerbate this loss and cause adverse effects on the ultimate processing of visual information. Once the light reaches the retina, that energy must be converted into a useful form that will convey information to the higher visual centers in the brain. How that energy is modified by the visual system is the subject of the following discussions.

Low-Level Visual Information Processing

There are at least two basic types of information in the visual environment that are processed by the retina. The first type is *spatial information*, which refers to the contour of the stimulus. Spatial information can also be regarded as a variation of luminance over a localized surface area. The second type of visual information can be regarded as *temporal information*, which refers either to changes of the stimulus's luminance content over time or to the processing that takes place with motion, as in the saccadic movement of the eyes during reading.

Although nomenclature may differ among authorities, there is good evidence of parallel processing for both spatial and temporal information in the retina.[16] Both types of information are processed simultaneously by separate mechanisms. Watching a movie is an analogy, in which sound is synchronized with pictures: Watching the film and listening to the sound involve separate mechanisms. As long as they remain in synchronization, what is seen and heard is optimally effective. Lack of synchronization of spatial and temporal visual information processing has an adverse effect on reading efficiency.

Retinal Process

To appreciate spatial and temporal processing, it is helpful to have a basic understanding of the mechanisms involved.
- Rod and cone cells provide basic wavelength (color) and luminance (brightness) information to the rest of the visual system.

- Cone cell output is modified by bipolar-horizontal cell interconnections (interaction). The result of these interactions is the formation of a receptive field. In turn, the output from this interaction serves as input to ganglion cells that transmit continuing color, contrast, and contour information.
- Cone cell output is also modified by bipolar-amacrine cell interaction, providing transient information to the ganglion cells related to rapid luminance change and motion.
- A portion of cone cell output is directed to extraretinocortical pathways, some of which terminate in the superior colliculus. Although not for sensory purposes, these pathways provide transient information related to motion detection.

Retinal Organization

Formation of the optical images of words on the retina sets the stage for initial visual information processing. This is the transformation of optical energy to electrochemical signals, called *phototransduction*. Although research has shown that cone cells are adapted for daylight and color information and rod cells are adapted for low light levels, retinal organization suggests a much greater degree of sophistication than can be expected from the output of these two types of photoreceptors.[17]

The retina is a stratified system whose ganglion cell output appears to be determined by the organization of the spatial and temporal information that precedes it. There are four divisions, or layers, within the retina that relate to the neural processing of information[18]: (1) the outer nuclear layer, which contains the cell bodies (perikarya) of the rods and cones; (2) the outer plexiform layer (OPL), which contains the dendrites of bipolar cells, the horizontal cell processes, and the cell terminals of the rods and cones, as well as processes from the interplexiform cells; (3) the inner nuclear layer, which contains the perikarya of the bipolar, horizontal, amacrine, and interplexiform cells; and (4) the inner plexiform layer (IPL), which contains the dendrites of the ganglion cells, the amacrine cell processes, the terminals of the bipolar cells, and the processes of the interplexiform cell.

Cell Processing for Spatial Information

Although relatively little is known about visual information processing in the scotopic (low light levels) rod system at photopic (high) light levels, abundant research has been conducted to clarify visual processing by cones. The cones have a graded, as opposed to an all-or-none, response to light. Factors include variations in intensity, color, and other features of light. Instead of typical depolarization at nerve terminals, the cone and rod response is a hyperpolarized one—that is, it becomes less active as the amount of light increases. For rod cells, as light intensity increases, the light response saturates under photopic conditions and for all practical purposes does not contribute to photopic response. Cone cells, however, do not fully saturate under normal photopic conditions and, thus, they remain active so reading can occur in normal illumination.

This type of graded response by the cones under photopic conditions is also present in the bipolar cells. The cone terminals synapse with the dendrites of two types of bipolar cells in the OPL. This segregation of two different types of synaptic connections, made by the bipolar cells, appears to signal the role the bipolar cells play in the transmission of spatial and temporal visual information.

Those bipolar cells, found *extrafoveally* and variously known as *on-center* response, depolarizing, or invaginating bipolar cells, have dendritic synapses within the invaginations of the cone cells. They generally appear to respond to sustained illumination, facilitating the excitation of ganglion cells.[18] The other type of bipolar cell, known as *off-center* response, hyperpolarizing, or flat bipolar, has its synaptic connections on the flattened base of the cone receptor terminals. This bipolar cell appears to transmit information that inhibits ganglion cell excitation with sustained illumination. Within the OPL, therefore, exists a mechanism to detect the static spatial aspects of brightness contrast. In other words, this is the detection of boundaries of light and dark where the neuronal comparisons form the basis of contrast information. Ganglion cells lend both excitatory and inhibitory signals to form a receptive field, organized in a circular center-surround fashion.

Although the center organization involves the cone-bipolar interaction, the surround field organization involves another cell that lies along the outer margin of the inner nuclear layer; this is the horizontal cell. The responses of bipolar or horizontal cells form the antagonistic center-surround organization that signals contrast detection. A networking adaptive mechanism is provided that can adjust its operating range on the basis of surround illumination.[18] Thus, the organization of the center response reflects a direct receptor-bipolar synaptic interaction, whereas the surround response appears to be mediated by horizontal cell activity.

The *foveal* area has a greater specialized functional organization than do other parts of the retina. Here, for the most part, each cone separates its sustained spatial information through synapses to bipolar cells known as midget bipolars (Figure 4.3). Their function appears to be similar to the extrafoveal bipolar cells associated with cone information. The output of the midget bipolars goes directly to dendrites from another class of specialized cells, called midget ganglion cells. These ganglion cells in the IPL maintain segregated spatial information from each, or possibly a few, bipolar cells. Some midget bipolar cells transmit excitatory ("on") information, whereas other midget bipolar cells transmit inhibitory ("off") information.

Some ganglion cell synapses within the IPL receive most of their input from the bipolar cells, which convey only sustained spatial activ-

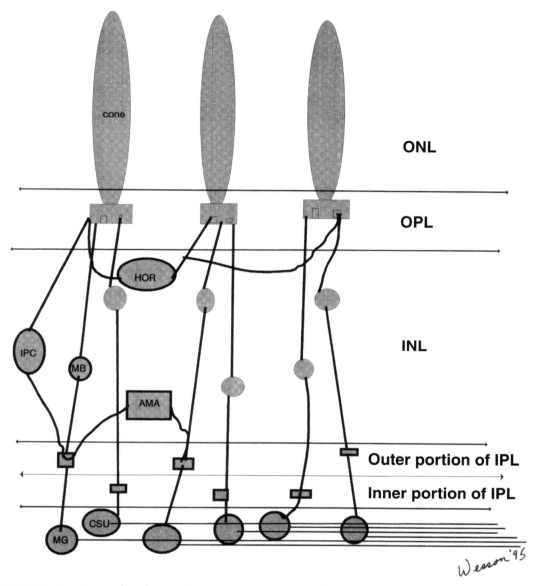

FIGURE 4.3 *Specialized synaptic interconnections within the foveal region for improved edge-detection capacity. (IPC = inner plexiform cell; MB = midget bipolar; MG = midget ganglion; AMA = amacrine cell; CSU = contrast sensitivity unit; HOR = horizontal cell; ONL = outer nuclear layer; OPL = outer plexiform layer; INL = inner nuclear layer; IPL = inner plexiform layer.)*

ity. This is a reflection of the type of visual information processing occurring in the OPL. As mentioned previously, processing in the OPL gives rise to the *spatial* processes in visual information. Output from these bipolar cells is routed to one type of ganglion cell, known as the contrast-sensitive unit, which is further subdivided into two mirror-image subunits, one with on-center activity and one with off-center activity.[18] The surround of the on-center subunit is antagonistic, and its stimulation causes a reduction (inhibition) of the activity of the sub-unit. On the other hand, when the center of the off-center subunit is illuminated, the cell's activity is inhibited. Stimulation of its surround, however, causes an increase in overall activity of the subunit. These cells are involved with the spatial information processing.

Transient Activity

Within the IPL there exists another cell class, known as the amacrine cell. There are two basic categories of amacrine cell activity: sustained and transient. Transient amacrine cell activity is responsive to moving stimuli.[18] In addition, when these cells receive information from a flickering light source, they display characteristics different from those of cells having a sustained function, such as horizontal and sustained amacrine cells.

Certain ganglion cells whose dendrites are in the IPL have been identified as receiving the majority, or possibly all, of their input from the amacrine cells. These ganglion cells initiate transient responses to be transmitted through the visual pathways.

Interplexiform Cells

Another retinal cell that deserves brief mention is the interplexiform cell.[18] This rather recently discovered cell appears to have connections to the two plexiform layers (OPL and IPL). Input to these cells comes exclusively from the amacrine cell processes in the IPL; output goes to the horizontal cells in the OPL. This means that information is being transmitted up to the outer layers (a centrifugal process), probably as a feedback system. Research indicates that these interplexiform cells help shape the center-surround organization of the receptive field and enhance the responsiveness of the bipolar cells.

Information Output from the Retina

The optics of the eye generate an MTF, which shapes the light signal input to the retina. A second MTF is generated by retinal processing, which further shapes the visual signal and serves as output to the reti-nal ganglion cells.

Ganglion Cell Activity

Retinal information output is reflected by activity in the axons of the retinal ganglion cells. In the cat, the majority of ganglion cell activity may be segregated into three distinct categories, which have been designated X and Y cells; there is another category called W cells.[19–21] The X cells behave in the same fashion as sustained on-center and off-center cells in the transfer of spatial information. The Y cells act as if they receive a mix of sustained spatial input (from bipolar cells) and transient temporal (from amacrine cells) input, resulting in the information transfer of luminance and motion.

It is tempting to carry this X and Y setup to humans. Although retinal ganglion cell activity in the primate has been sorted into cell classes, there is no strong evidence for the same type of X-Y organization.[22–24] A more widely accepted classification divides the ganglion cells into two broad classes, P and M, as a function of their connections to the lateral geniculate nucleus (LGN).[17, 25]

P and M Cell Classification

The P cell is a small ganglion cell whose axons connect within the upper four layers of the LGN, which are the parvocellular layers.[17] The receptive fields from the P cells are small, with well-organized center-surrounds, and they are color opponent. Color opponency refers to cone output through the bipolar cells mediated by the horizontal cells. The resulting response is based on wavelength preference. For example, the center of the receptive field may be red-excitatory and the surround, green-inhibitory. Research corroborates this type of organization within the foveal area of the primate retina. With this type of receptive field organization, color, contrast, and edge detection information may be transmitted by the same mechanism. The human P cell relays essentially the same type of *spatial-sustained* information to the LGN as that carried by the ganglion cells found in the cat.

The M cell has a larger cell body than the P cell, and its axons connect with layers 5 and 6 of the LGN (the magnocellular layers).[17] The receptive fields of this cell are larger than those of the P cell, and the center-surround organization reflects input of more than one cone type (red, green, and blue) into the antagonistic field organization. Combinations of all three cone types appear to transmit luminosity as well as *temporal-transient* information.[17]

Retinal Output to the Superior Colliculus

Another ganglion cell, of which little is known, is found in the primate retina. There is some suggestion that this cell is like the W cell of the cat and includes about 10% of the retinal output. This output terminates in the superior colliculus.[17] There are three general subdivisions of the superior colliculus: the superficial, intermediate, and deep layers. The superficial layers of the colliculus receive input directly from the retinal periphery as well as indirect input from the ipsilateral visual cortex. The retinal information is of a short-latency, high-velocity, transient nature. Consequently, the fibers relaying this information are highly sensitive to rapid-stimulus onset-offset (flicker) and motion.

Visual Cortex

Based on morphologic, physiologic, and psychophysical evidence, parallel processing of visual information from the retina to the LGN appears also to continue to the visual cortex (area 17). The magnocellular layers of the LGN project to layer 4C alpha and then to the middle temporal cortical area. The parvocellular layers project to 4C beta, then to layers 2 and 3 as well as to adjacent cortical areas.[26] In the LGN, the parvocellular system is characterized by color opponency, low contrast sensitivity, and high spatial resolution. The magnocellular system displays high contrast sensitivity, fast temporal resolution, and low spatial resolution.

Livingstone and Hubel[27] suggested that within the cortex the magnocellular and parvocellular systems further divide to become the magno, parvo-interblob, and blob systems. The magno system is related to movement sensitivity, fast temporal resolution, and low spatial resolution. The parvo-interblob system exhibits low contrast sensitivity, slow temporal resolution, and high spatial resolution. The parvo-interblob system appears to be important for fine detail discrimination as well as other specific properties. The functions of the blob system are less well defined and are not discussed in this text.

Ergonomic Aspects

An excellent review of ergonomics of reading and visual information processing is covered by Garzia.[28] In addition to discussions of the factors of lighting and typography, consideration is given to special issues of reading from video display terminals (VDTs). Prescribing the optimal refractive correction, including near addition lenses, is important when managing complaints associated with VDT use. The design of near addition lenses is a critical factor in addressing visual task requirements, including consideration of size, shape, and placement. VDTs also place significant demands on the accommodative and vergence systems, resulting in a high percentage of symptoms related to binocular vision disorders. A thorough evaluation of vision efficiency skills, as discussed in Chapter 9, is recommended for VDT users. Management of symptoms may include a program of vision therapy to improve deficient visual efficiency skills. It is important to assist the patient in evaluating the ergonomics of the computer workstation. This should include assessment of lighting characteristics; screen glare and reflections; positioning of keyboard, screen and chair; and posture during computer use.

Summary

Type size, print contrast, and light source considerations are important physical aspects of the reading process. Some spatial and temporal processing occurs at the level of the retina through modification of cone cell output and interaction of the bipolar and amacrine cells. Retinal output is segregated into spatial (parvocellular) and temporal (magnocellular) information channels. Further evidence of this mechanism for parallel processing is shown in the retino-geniculo-calcarine pathway. Understanding of these physical and physiologic processes provides the groundwork for discussion in subsequent chapters on clinical implications of visual processing deficits.

References

1. Vellutino FR, Pruzek RM, Steger JA, et al. Intermediate visual recall in poor and normal readers as a function of age and orthographic-linguistic familiarity. Cortex 1973;9:370–86.
2. Vellutino FR, Steger JA, Kamin M, et al. Visual form perception in deficient and normal readers as a function of age and oto-linguistic familiarity. Cortex 1975;11:22–30.
3. Vellutino FR, Steger JA, Harding CJ, et al. Verbal vs. non-verbal paired-associates learning in poor and normal readers. Neuropsychologia 1975;13:75–82.
4. Fisher DF, Frankfurter A. Normal and disabled readers can locate and identify letters: where's the perceptual deficit? J Read Behav 1977;10:31–43.
5. Morrison F, Giordani B, Nagy J. Reading disability: an information processing analysis. Science 1977;196:77–9.
6. Arnett JL, DiLollo V. Visual information processing in relation to age and to reading ability. J Exp Child Psychol 1979;27:143–52.
7. Hulme C. The implausibility of low-level visual deficits as a cause of children's reading difficulty. Neurophysiol 1988;5:369–74.
8. Manny RE, Fern KD, Loshin DS. Contour interaction function in the preschool child. Am J Optom Physiol Optics 1987;64:686–92.
9. Flom MC, Heath GC, Takahashi E. Contour interaction and visual resolution: contralateral effects. Science 1963;142:979–80.
10. Flom MC, Weymouth FW, Kahneman D. Visual resolution and contour interaction. J Opt Soc Am 1963;53:1026–32.
11. Davidson DW. Design and clinical evaluation of a psychometric test of visual acuity for amblyopic patients. University of Alabama at Birmingham, Master's Thesis 1975.
12. Robson JG. Neural Images: The Physiological Basis of Spatial Vision. In CS Harris (ed), Visual Coding and Adaptability. Hillsdale, NJ: Lawerence Erlbaum, 1980;177–214.
13. Marr D. Vision: A Computational Investigation into the Human Representation and Processing of Visual Information. San Francisco: Freeman, 1982;61–74.

14. Cornsweet T. Visual Perception. New York: Academic, 1970.
15. Ball K, Owsley C, Sloane M. Visual and cognitive predictors of driving problems in older adults. Exp Aging Res 1991;17:79–80.
16. Bassi CJ. Parallel Processing In the Human Visual System. In M Wall, AA Sedun (eds), New Methods of Sensory Visual Testing. New York: Springer-Verlag, 1989;1–13.
17. Miller RF. The Physiology and Morphology of the Vertebrate Retina. In TE Ogden (ed), Retina. St. Louis: Mosby 1989;1:83–106.
18. Dowling JE. The Retina: An Approachable Part of the Brain. Cambridge MA: Belnap Press, 1987.
19. Enroth-Cugell C, Robson JG. The contrast sensitivity of retinal ganglion cells of the cat. J Physiol (Lond) 1966;187:517–52.
20. Peichl L, Wassle H. Morphological identification of on-and off-center brisk transient (Y) cells in the cat retina. Proc R Soc Lond Biol Sci 1981;212:139–56.
21. Peichl L, Wassle H. The structural correlate of the receptive field center of alpha ganglion cells in the cat retina. J Physiol (Lond) 1983;341:309–24.
22. DeMonasterio FM. Properties of concentrically organized X- and Y-ganglion cells of the macaque retina. J Neurophysiol 1978;41:1435–49.
23. Gouras PJ. Identification of cone mechanisms in monkey ganglion cells. J Physiol (Lond) 1968;199:533–47.
24. Schiller PH, Malpeli JG. Functional specificity of lateral geniculate nucleus laminae of the rhesus monkey. J Neurophysiol 1978;41:788–97.
25. Shapley RM, Perry VH. Cat and monkey retinal ganglion cells and their functional roles. Trends Neurosci 1986;9:229–35.
26. Wall M, Sedun AA (eds). New Methods of Sensory Visual Testing. New York: Springer-Verlag, 1989;2.
27. Livingstone MS, Hubel DH. Psychophysical evidence for separate channels for the perception of form, color, movement and depth. J Neurosci 1987;7:3416–68.
28. Garzia RP (ed). Vision and Reading. Mosby's Optometric Problem-Solving Series. St. Louis: Mosby, 1996.

5 Low-Level Visual Processing Deficits

The transient system (magno-interblob) appears to be defective in a subpopulation with reading dysfunction (RD), and this transient system visual deficit can be detected by using psychophysical methods. What follows is a description of representative studies discussing the nature of this deficit. Samplings of experimental designs are presented to give an overview of the type of research being performed in this area. Most of the experimental and laboratory procedures are omitted for the sake of brevity.

Visual Deficit Hypothesis

The presence of visual processing deficits in poor readers—that is, readers with RD—was apparently first proposed by Bryant.[1] Experimental evidence supporting this concept was cited as early as 1976 by Clifton-Everest.[2] Other proponents are cited in the following discussions, but the deficit hypothesis has been challenged by Vellutino et al.,[3–5] Fisher and Frankfurter,[6] Morrison et al.,[7] Arnett and Di Lollo,[8] and Hulme.[9] As we shall see, however, perusal of the more recent literature clearly supports the presence of a low-level (i.e., occurring early in the visual process before cognition) visual information–processing deficit in a subpopulation of poor readers. This deficit, revealed in several experimental paradigms, appears to be related to the processing of temporal (often referred to as transient) information early in the visual information–processing sequence. Brietmeyer and Ganz[10] proposed that temporal processing can occur either at the beginning of the retinal process (in the retina) or in the visual cortex. Some investigators refer to these processing locations as peripheral (retina) and central (cortical). These terms should not be confused with central retina versus peripheral retina. The important implication is that this type of visual processing occurs without the need for higher-order cognitive function.

Visual Processing Deficits and Cognitive Function

The nature of the psychophysical task is crucial in any experiment attempting to differentiate normal from poor readers. The usual definition of a poor reader is one who is reading 2 or more years below grade placement. As will be pointed out in Chapter 6, the value of visual-perceptual-motor (VPM) testing and evaluation in cases of RD is evident. Nevertheless, traditional VPM tests using isolated spatial arrays presented for relatively long periods of time (possibly several seconds or even untimed) do not provide substantive evidence for predicting specific RD. This conclusion is in accord with the results of Vellutino et al.[3–5] and others who have performed this type of experimental paradigm involving visual motor and visual memory tasks. All these tasks appear to be mediated by perceptual processing, which requires *higher-level cognitive* demands. In some visual experiments, however, *low-level, noncognitive* visual processing deficits have been revealed in poor readers. The following discussion of a selected sample of experimental studies illustrates that low-level (preattentive) temporal deficits are present in the visual information processing system of at least some poor readers.

Low-Level Temporal Processing Deficits

Most of the visual information processing differences between good and poor readers have been found to involve low-level visual processing in the temporal domain. Samples of psychophysical investigations that have uncovered low-level deficits in the temporal domain include (1) short-duration or successive stimuli presentation,[11–14] (2) temporal resolution,[15, 16] (3) visible persistence duration (VPD),[14, 17–21] (4) flicker masking effects[22, 23] and temporal contrast sensitivity,[24–27] (5) perceptual grouping[28] and visual search,[29–31] and (6) transient system modification.[32, 33] These and other areas of investigation are summarized here, illustrating the effect of low-level visual processing in the temporal domain. Each section is accompanied by a table outlining the salient points of the experiments described in that section.

Successive Stimuli and Short-Duration Presentation

The following studies illustrate the strong interaction effect of briefly presented, successive stimuli (Table 5.1).

Stanley and Hall (1973)

Stanley and Hall[11] in this and other related studies[12, 13] compared the early stages of visual information processing in subjects with and without RD using a successive stimulus paradigm. The subjects were 66 children, divided into two matched groups: those with RD and a control group. The children with RD were differentiated from the control group by the following criteria: (1) "specific reading disability" of 2.5 years below normal, (2) performance at average or better levels in other academic subjects, (3) absence of gross behavioral problems, and (4) absence of organic disorders (these criteria are more or less typical of all the studies evaluated in this chapter and form the basis of most comparison studies of normal readers with those with RD). The control subjects were selected by their class teachers as "average to

TABLE 5.1   Low-Level Visual Processing Deficits Probed with Successive Short-Duration Stimuli

Authors	Year	Objective of Research into Visual Processing Differences Between Normal and Poor Readers (RDs)	Research Method	Results
Stanley and Hall	1973	To determine low-level visual processing differences	Successive, short duration half-figure presentations with increasing time intervals (ISIs)	RDs required larger ISIs to identify figures (possible temporal integration deficit)
Lovegrove and Brown	1978	To determine visual information-store duration differences in two age groups for presence of maturational factor	Establish ISIs for two age groups using method of Stanley and Hall (1973)	Apparent maturational influence noted
Lyle and Goyen	1975	To determine low-level temporal integration and visual discrimination differences	Consecutive, short-term tachistoscopic exposures of geometric figures	RDs required longer tachistoscopic exposure times to recognize figures

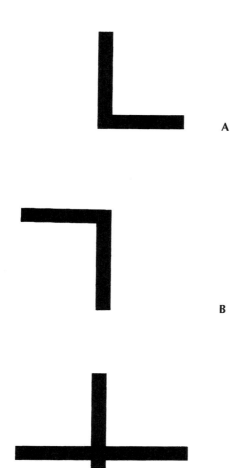

FIGURE 5.1 *Stimuli used by Stanley and Hall. A. Half-figure (L-shaped target). B. Half-figure (inverted L-shaped target). C. Composite figure. (From G Stanley, R Hall. Short-term visual information processing in dyslexics. Child Dev 1973;44:841–4.)*

bright students." For each group, the age range was 8–12 years, with a mean age of approximately 10.5 years.

In the first of two experiments, two half-figures were briefly presented either at the same time or with varied interstimulus intervals (ISIs) between presentations. The subject's task was to report when the two half-figures could be identified as separate. For example, the investigators presented two targets that together formed a plus symbol. As the time interval between presentations of the two half-figures was increased in 20-millisecond steps, a point was reached at which the subject was able to recognize the figure as being composed of two parts: an L-shaped target and an inverted L–shaped target (Figure 5.1). The subject accomplished this task by drawing or describing each part.

In the second experiment, familiar letters (i.e., previously identified by the subjects) were flashed on a screen, followed by a masking stimulus in the same spatial location presented 20 milliseconds after the letter. The masking stimulus, at the same spatial locus of the prior letter stimulus, acted to interfere with the perception of the previously presented letter (this is known as *backward masking*). The ISIs of the mask were increased by 20-millisecond steps until three correct responses were given.

The experimental results of this investigation demonstrated significant visual processing differences between those with RD and normal readers. In the first experiment, children with RD required significantly longer ISIs to identify a separation of the half-figures ($p < 0.01$). In the second experiment, the RD group took significantly longer ($p < 0.01$) to identify the letters in the backward masking design. These two experiments suggest that people with RD may manifest visual-temporal integration problems and require longer processing time than normal readers and that the processing problems occur early in the analysis of the stimulus by the visual system.

Lovegrove and Brown (1978)

Lovegrove and Brown[14] investigated an aspect of temporal integration by measuring visual information–store duration for normal and poor readers, whom they labeled dyslexic. Although they defined dyslexics as being 2 years below the appropriate reading level for their age, with normal intelligence and no known gross organic disorders or behavioral problems, we will refer to these subjects as having RD for clarity.

Visual information–store duration, which we will call visual persistence duration (VPD), refers to a low-level visual process similar to that investigated by Stanley and Hall.[11] Two brief (20-millisecond) stimuli are presented in succession until, by shortening ISI, the two appear to be present at the same time (the briefer the ISI, the better the integrative process). Lovegrove and Brown's experiments were designed to examine whether age and the presence of RD affected VPD. The results showed that the ISI was significantly longer for the younger groups than for the older groups. For both age groups, however, subjects with RD displayed a 30% longer ISI. This suggests that temporal integration was deficient in the RD group when compared with the controls. There was no significant difference when the average ISI for the older RD group was compared to the younger controls. This result implies that the difference was one of maturation—that is, the older RD group was processing visual information at the same rate as the younger control group of normal readers.

Temporal Resolution (Lyle and Goyen, 1975)

Lyle and Goyen[15] took a different approach in a series of experiments, the first of which was published in 1968.[16] Subjects with RD performed less well on tachistoscopic exposure tasks than did normal readers. Tachistoscopic exposure refers to briefly presented visual stimuli flashed on a screen (usually letters, numbers, or geometric figures). Lyle and Goyen were interested in answering questions of whether people with RD manifest a low-level temporal integration problem (although they did not refer to their results in those terms), whether people with RD have some form of visual discrimination problem primarily related to the difficulty of discriminating alternatives on response cards, or whether there is a defect in short-term visual memory. They answered these questions in a relatively straightforward experiment later in their series.[15]

Lyle and Goyen speculated that the evidence accumulated over this series of experiments suggested a maturational effect. That is, up to about 8.5 years of age, the differences between reading groups were clear. Beyond that age, however, it was their opinion that verbal and intellectual factors tended to obscure the differences.

Visible Persistence Duration

Five studies of the VPD are presented in this section (Table 5.2).

Lovegrove, Billing, and Slaghuis (1978)

In a set of experiments published in the same year as those of Lovegrove and Brown,[14] VPD and contour orientation information processing in the visual cortex were investigated by Lovegrove, Billing, and Slaghuis.[17] They were aware that many individuals with RD confused letters with similar orientation components, as reported by other investigators.[34, 35] They reasoned that, if orientation effects could be localized at different levels within the visual system, the locus for the orientation dysfunction might be uncovered through measures of VPD.

Their results supported those of Stanley and Hall[11] with respect to VPD differences between subjects with RD and normal readers: Those with RD have visual-temporal integration problems.

Lovegrove, Heddle, and Slaghuis (1980)

Lovegrove, Heddle, and Slaghuis[18] studied the temporal response differences between normal and poor readers by assessing VPD at various spatial frequencies by measuring children's responses to gratings (light and dark stripes) with high contrast. At higher spatial frequencies, the temporal-spatial interaction was less robust. This reduced the difference in VPD between the RD group and normal readers. Other investigations have corroborated these results.[22, 37–41]

TABLE 5.2 Effect of the Duration of Visible Persistence in the Spatial Domain on Low-Level Visual Processing

Authors	Year	Objective of Research into Visual Processing Differences Between Normal and Poor Readers (RDs)	Research Method	Results
Lovegrove, Billing, and Slaghuis	1978	To determine if contour orientation information together with visual information–store (VIS) duration differentially affected reading groups	3-channel tachistoscope with line pairs of different orientation	Processing differences probably cortical rather than retinal
Lovegrove, Heddle, and Slaghuis	1980	To determine the difference in VIS duration using spatial contrast sensitivity with 8-year-olds	3-channel tachistoscope with spatial gratings in 2 channels and space-averaged blank field in third channel	Differential response noted at lower spatial frequencies
Lovegrove, Bowling, Badcock, and Black-wood	1981	To determine the difference in VIS duration using spatial contrast sensitivity with 14-year-olds	3-channel tachistoscope with varied spatial frequencies, exposure times, and contrast levels	Apparent cortical processing time differences permit contrast sensitivity curves to be established 5–10 times faster in normal readers
Badcock and Lovegrove	1981	To investigate visual sensitivity differences between younger and older children using spatial contrast sensitivity	3-channel tachistoscope with varied spatial frequencies, exposure times, and contrast levels	Visual processing differences remain in older children, indicating the effect is not maturational but sensory
Slaghuis and Lovegrove	1984	Investigated differences in spatial-temporal interaction through temporal (i.e., flicker) masking	3-channel tachistoscope with varied spatial frequencies and temporal (6-Hz) mask	Demonstrated temporal defect in RDs and provided additional evidence for Breitmeyer's hypothesis

Lovegrove, Bowling, Badcock, and Blackwood (1980)

Although VPD provides a measure of temporal processing, there is evidence that the differences between readers with RD and normal readers are also manifest in certain measures of spatial contrast sensitivity. This hypothesis was tested by Lovegrove et al.,[21] who investigated differences in visual sensitivity found in grating presentations at various spatial frequencies between readers with RD and normal readers.

For both groups tested at presentations of 100 milliseconds or less, contrast thresholds for all frequencies increased (decrease in sensitivity) as the exposure time became shorter. When the presentations were longer than 100 milliseconds, the control group began to develop the typical bandpass function associated with contrast sensitivity curves, with a maximum sensitivity appearing at 4 cycles per degree (cpd). However, the RD subjects did not display such a peak until exposure times reached 1,000 milliseconds. Bowling and Lovegrove[40, 41] suggested that cortical processing differences, as opposed to retinal processing differences, between the two groups were responsible for these results. These results certainly support differences in temporal processing between normal readers and those with RD.

Interestingly, the stimulus durations that produce the greatest difference between the two groups are at the same duration as most saccadic eye movement durations in reading (150–200 milliseconds), providing additional evidence for the Breitmeyer model of transient-on-sustained inhibition.[10]

Badcock and Lovegrove (1981)

In 1981, Badcock and Lovegrove[19] reported the effects of contrast, stimulus duration, and spatial frequency on VPD in normal readers and subjects with RD using a different paradigm. The subjects were 24 children, divided into two groups of 12 with an average age of 14.3 years and an average IQ of 100. The investigators wanted to know if older subjects with RD displayed the same deficiencies found in the younger RD subjects with respect to the VPD at specific spatial frequencies.[18] In other words, is the observed effect one of maturation or the result of a sensory deficit?

As with other experiments, the RD group exhibited significantly longer VPDs at low spatial frequencies.[18] In both groups, with increasing spatial frequency, the VPD increased (i.e., performance became worse), but the slope of the curve for the controls was significantly steeper. These results indicated that, for the older population (i.e., 14-year-olds vs. 8-year-olds), differences between normal readers and those with RD continue to exist. This runs counter to the proposal by Fletcher and Satz[42] and Lyle and Goyen[15] that this deficit would be present only in the younger population. Statistical analysis indicated that the differences were not based on the use of differing response criteria, for which earlier studies have been criticized.

Evidence exists that there is a sequence from general visual information processing (related to low spatial frequencies) to detailed visual processing (high spatial frequencies).[43] Subjects with RD in this study showed markedly different temporal patterns across spatial frequencies with different stimulus durations. The most aberrant patterns were displayed at stimulus durations that came close to the saccadic durations normally found in the act of reading. Breitmeyer and Ganz[10] and Breitmeyer[44] expanded on the concept of Vienet et al.,[45] proposing that reading involves a narrow range of spatial frequencies interacting with the temporal processing of visual information, which is referred to as *temporal-on-sustained inhibition*. In the act of reading, this inhibition terminates visible persistence from a prior fixation. If this did not occur, forward masking would blur the next fixation.

Another way of discussing this issue relates to peripheral versus central processing. It is possible that two components of visual persistence exist: peripheral (retinal) and central (cortical). Short-duration stimuli elicit responses in both peripheral and central processing, whereas longer-duration stimuli elicit only cortical responses. Differences in response characteristics between the RD group and normal readers to low-contrast spatial gratings support a central processing difference, but not a peripheral difference. This would explain the findings of other researchers,[8, 46, 47] in which retinal VPD was measured and no difference found between RD subjects and normal readers. These results suggest that the differences in VPD between people with RD and normal readers occur primarily in the cortex, not in the retina.

Returning to Breitmeyer's hypothesis,[10] the faster-acting, low-frequency channels serve as a guide for retinal information during reading. If the RD subject cannot use this low-frequency information, erratic eye movements may occur (see Chapter 7 for information on eye movements and RD).

Slaghuis and Lovegrove (1984)

Slaghuis and Lovegrove[22] investigated differences between people with RD and normal readers in the transient system by evaluation of the VPD using spatial frequency channels masked by a temporal stimulus (i.e., 6-Hz flicker).

When the 6-Hz mask was not present, the control group displayed a proportional increase in the VPD with increasing spatial frequency. The RD group, however, showed no difference from the controls at spatial frequencies under 4 cpd, but had significantly shorter VPD at frequencies of 4 cpd and higher, with a slope of about half that of the normal readers.

In the presence of the 6-Hz flicker mask, the effect on the control group was to increase significantly the VPD at low spatial frequencies compared to the unmasked condition. At higher spatial frequencies, however, there was a differential effect as the normal readers displayed a negligible change in VPD and the RD group's VPD increased significantly. The overall result was that, under masked conditions, there were no apparent differences between the RD group and controls over all spatial frequencies tested.

These results confirm other studies[19, 48] that demonstrate that VPD is greater for readers with RD than for controls with decreasing spatial frequencies within a limited range. This study also indicates that when flicker (6 Hz) was used as a temporal mask, Breitmeyer, Levi, and Harweth's[23] hypothesis is supported. That is, the presence of a temporal stimulus (i.e., the 6-Hz mask) significantly increased VPD for the controls at low spatial frequencies but had only a relatively small effect on the RD subjects at these same spatial frequencies. The fact that the RD subjects were not as influenced by the mask at low spatial frequencies indicates that, under normal conditions, they had very little transient-on-sustained inhibition. This can be interpreted to mean that people with RD do not have much of a temporal system to inhibit. At low spatial frequencies, therefore, no significant changes were noted.

Flicker Masking and Temporal Contrast Sensitivity Differences

Up to this point we have focused on differences of a temporal nature between normal readers and those with RD. These differences, however, have been couched in psychophysical paradigms that have both spatial and temporal properties. Psychophysical methods exist that use a much purer form of temporal measurement, which is related to flicker and contrast of the flickering field (i.e., a homogeneous flickering field), referred to as the temporal contrast sensitivity function (TCSF) (De Lange function[49]) (Figure 5.2). Following is a selection of experiments illustrating the use of the TCSF as a tool for separating those with RD from normal readers. In some of these experiments, only full-field flicker is used to determine the TCSF. Others use some spatial measure for TCSF measurement (Table 5.3).

Martin and Lovegrove (1984, 1987)

Martin and Lovegrove[24, 25] used the TCSF in examining low-level visual processing in the temporal system of RD subjects. Their objective in a representative experimental paradigm[25] was to ascertain whether there were differences in the TCSF between normal readers and those with RD. The TCSF is obtained by using a flickering homogeneous stimulus having *temporal* frequencies (in Hz) that can be varied with contrast. The RD group displayed reduced contrast sensitivity at all temporal fre-

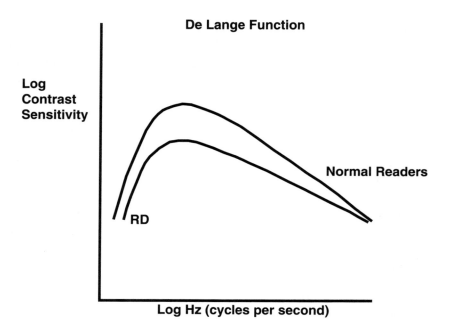

FIGURE 5.2 *De Lange (temporal contrast sensitivity) function. The graph is pictured on a log-log scale with the x-axis in cycles per second (Hz) and the y-axis plotted as the inverse of contrast threshold (contrast sensitivity). (RD = subjects with reading dysfunction.)*

quencies, with the greatest contrast sensitivity losses at higher temporal frequencies.

They also investigated the effect of holding a high temporal frequency constant (at 20 Hz) and measuring the contrast sensitivity of a series of gratings whose spatial frequency was varied from 1 cpd to 12 cpd. The subjects with RD were again less sensitive than the controls at all spatial frequencies tested, with the difference increasing toward higher spatial frequencies.

The results suggest that RD subjects are significantly less sensitive than normal readers in temporal processing. In addition, the deficit in the transient system appeared to occur at an early level of visual processing. Therefore, it most likely influences processing at any subsequent level.

Brannan and Williams (1988)

Brannan and Williams[26] have also investigated flicker thresholds between normal readers and those with RD at three age levels with adults as controls. The results indicated a clear developmental trend for flicker threshold—that is, the older children displayed better temporal sensitivity than the younger children in both the normal reading group

TABLE 5.3 Temporal Contrast Sensitivity Differences Between Normal Readers and Those with Reading Dysfunction (RDs)

Authors	Year	Objective of Research into Visual Processing Differences Between Normal and RDs	Research Method	Results
Martin and Lovegrove	1987	To use the temporal contrast sensitivity function (TCSF) to examine low-level visual processing differences	Counter-phase flicker of spatial frequency grating (2 cpd) at different temporal frequencies and varying contrast levels	RDs displayed reduced temporal contrast sensitivity at all temporal frequencies
Brannan and Williams	1987	To investigate age effects using the TCSF	Full-field, homogeneous flicker at 6 temporal frequencies	Revealed a sensory deficit in the temporal domain, rather than a maturational lag
Martin and Lovegrove	1988	To investigate the impact of full-field flicker as a mask when imposed on spatial frequency channels	Low- and high-frequency full-field flicker was imposed on stationary spatial gratings of changing contrast	No difference in sensory response in the presence of full-field flicker

cpd = cycles per degree.

and the RD group. When the 12-year-old normal readers were compared to adults, the normal readers were not significantly different from the adults with respect to temporal sensitivity. Those with RD were significantly different from adults and from the normal readers in their respective age groups. This was especially true for lower temporal frequencies (4, 8, and 12 Hz). Based on this information, it appears that the etiology is a sensory deficit rather than maturational lag.

To strengthen this position, when older children who were reading at lower levels were matched with younger children who were reading at age-appropriate levels, the younger children who were normal readers displayed better temporal sensitivity than the older children with RD. This evidence again supports a true sensory difference rather than a maturational delay.

Martin and Lovegrove (1988)

Martin and Lovegrove provided further evidence for a temporal sensitivity deficit.[27] The objective in their experimental paradigm was to determine the effect of uniform-field flicker (6 Hz and 20 Hz) as a mask on stationary gratings at five spatial frequencies on temporal processing in normal and RD readers. Their data suggest that a significant correlation exists between flicker thresholds and reading level. This compares favorably with the investigation of Brannan and Williams[30] that found that flicker threshold accounted for 58% of the unique reading level variance when multiple regression analysis was used between flicker threshold, reading level, and age.

The experiments of Martin and Lovegrove[27] and others provide strong support for a deficit in the transient system of RD. The deficits found in these experiments may also have an adverse effect on higher-level visual processing, such as visual search and perceptual grouping tasks.[28, 32]

Perceptual Grouping and Visual Search

Perceptual grouping refers to linking segments of visual elements into figures and regions. This process takes place very early in the visual-perceptual sequence. Gestalt psychologists demonstrated that, when similar elements were grouped in close spatial proximity, those elements become part of the same perceptual unit. Actual evidence comes from Pomerantz and colleagues.[50, 51]

Williams and Bologna (1985)

Williams and Bologna[28] suggested that reading requires the use of perceptual grouping at the initial stages in the visual-perceptual sequence. They theorized that perceptual grouping is associated with transient

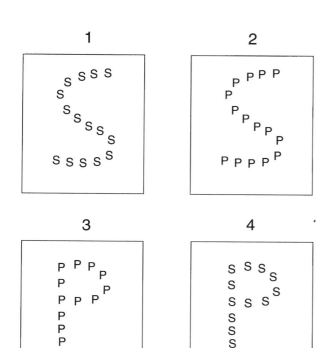

FIGURE 5.3 *Card sorting routine. Subjects with reading dysfunction (RD) tended to match by perceptual grouping rather than by matching details. For example, RD subjects would be more likely than normal readers to identify cards 1 and 2 as the same.*

activity, as first suggested by Williams and Weisstein.[52] Using the procedure developed by Pomerantz, they investigated perceptual grouping differences between readers 1 year above their expected reading level and those 1 year below level. The experiments involved card sorting routines (Figure 5.3). It is beyond the scope of this chapter to explore the details of the sorting tasks. Sorting time data, however, demonstrated that poor readers show stronger perceptual grouping effects than good readers do. In fact, as reading ability declines, the perceptual grouping effect increases. The conclusion was that poor readers are less proficient at selective attention to elements within a "perceptual unit." Failure of selective attention implies that visual information is processed more like a whole or unit. The peripheral information process is thought of as holistic and functions as an early warning system for analysis of incoming extramacular information. This peripheral process is considered preattentive (without conscious control). In essence, the poor reader is less able to exert active control over reading behavior and is relatively limited to a preattentive mode for visual processing.

Williams and Bologna suggest that this holistic process affects decoding by forcing the poor reader into "locking onto an early percept of the word."[28] Thus, the poor reader obtains the initial sound of the first few letters and is not able to process the remainder of the word.

The results of another investigation[29] also support this holistic concept. Using temporal-order stimuli, May, Williams, and Dunlop found that individuals with RD require more time to make a judgment about the temporal order than they needed to judge the spatial position of two briefly presented stimuli. Allocation of attention to different aspects of the stimuli may have contributed to this difference, and their data lend support to this position as well as to the position that process occurs early in the sensory (i.e., visual) mechanism. (Refer to Table 5.4.)

Brannan and Williams (1987)

Brannan and Williams[30] also investigated allocation of visual attention in normal and poor readers. Their method was to present cue information to help predict where a letter would appear on a video display terminal (VDT). This cue information was a line that suddenly appeared on the VDT providing early information for predicting the location of a letter to be flashed on the screen. The results suggested that poor readers do not use cue information efficiently in a temporal order task. Normal readers, on the other hand, were able to allocate visual attention across different points in space (across the face of the VDT) without the use of eye movements by taking advantage of cue information. This strategy is referred to as *analytic*. Subjects with RD were unable to use this form of allocation effectively in temporal order judgments and were judged to be operating in the "holistic" (preattentive) mode.

Brannan and Williams also reported that normal readers had a right visual field bias. That is, the identification of letters following cue information was more accurate when the right hemifield was stimulated. RD subjects did not show a bias for either right or left hemifield. We suggest a possible explanation for this observation. It is well established that speech and language centers are located in the left cerebral hemisphere for the large majority of individuals. The most direct route for visual information to these language centers is via the right visual hemifield. This may explain the bias in nondyslexic individuals. Dyslexics, however, are thought to have neurologic problems in the brain's language centers and, thus, the bias would possibly be less distinct compared with nondyslexic individuals.

Brannan and Williams (1988)

In an extension of the Williams and Bologna study,[28] Brannan and Williams[31] investigated the effect of maturation on perceptual grouping in normal readers and those with RD. Using both card sorting tasks and temporal order and position stimuli, they found that normal readers were better at all tasks for each age group. In addition, the time

TABLE 5.4   Differences Between Normal Readers and those with Reading Dysfunction (RDs) in Perceptual Grouping and Visual Search

Authors	Year	Objective of Research into Visual Processing Differences Between Normal Readers and RDs	Research Method	Results
Williams and Bologna	1985	To investigate perceptual grouping (PG) differences	Timed card sorting	Significant differences in PG: as reading skills decline, PG effect increases
Brannan and Williams	1987	To investigate how cue information is used in temporal order (i.e., sequential) tasks without the use of eye movements	Short-duration video-display cues flashed "off-fixation" to be used as location predictor	RDs unable to use cue information effectively in temporally ordered tasks
Brannan and Williams	1988	To investigate maturation-related PG	Timed card sorting tasks in 8-, 10-, and 12-year-olds	Good readers better at all tasks for every age group but maturational effects unsupported
Williams, Brannan, and Lartigue	1987	To investigate visual search using clear and blurred stimuli to see if high spatial frequency reduction affected RD performance	Scanning letter arrays for target letter with and without blur (from frosted acetate)	Differences between RDs and normal readers eliminated by stimulus blur
Williams, Lecluyse, and Rock-Faucheux	1992	To investigate "global" versus "detailed" visual information processing	Measured reading ability of RDs and normal readers through different colored filters and image blur	Differences between RDs and normal readers eliminated by stimulus blur and specific color (blue)

needed to complete the tasks decreased as age increased for both normal and poor readers.

Does this reduction in task completion time with age signal that a maturational effect might be responsible for the measured differences between normal and poor readers? The evidence cited in this investigation does not support the maturation hypothesis. When the older (10- or 12-year-old) children with RD were matched with younger (8- or 10-year-old) normal readers, the normal readers continued to exhibit better (smaller) perceptual grouping effects. This result strongly argues *against* a maturational effect and supports a fundamental processing difference between normal and poor readers.

Transient System Modification

Williams, Brannan, and Lartigue (1987)

Visual search tasks can also signal temporal processing differences. These differences are moderated when the image is blurred slightly from a normally clear image to assist in compensating for the dysfunction of the temporal system.

Williams, Brannan, and Lartigue[32] used such a visual search task for normal and poor readers under conditions of both clear and blurred visual arrays (i.e., the contrast of high spatial frequencies was reduced). Their subjects consisted of 10 children from 8 to 10 years old, divided into five "good" readers (1 year above grade level) and five "poor" readers (1 year below grade level). Each stimulus array, which was presented for an unlimited time, was made up of 16 rows of letters with six letters in each row. One of the letters in each row was a target letter (the letter Z) (Figure 5.4). It was the subject's task to scan the rows as quickly as he or she could and press a buzzer when the target letter was located.

With clear stimuli, the search time for the normal readers was substantially better than that of the poor readers. With blurred high spatial frequencies, however, the difference between poor and normal readers disappeared.

The high spatial frequencies seem to be associated with a sensory deficit because the response time of the poor readers improved when the visual arrays were presented slightly out of focus. The blur had no effect on normal readers. The investigators hypothesized that blurring the high spatial frequencies slows the sustained system so that the more sluggish transient system of readers with RD is able once again to establish its temporal precedence.

Williams, Lecluyse, and Rock-Faucheux (1992)

Williams, Lecluyse, and Rock-Faucheux[33] extended the concept that there are two separate but interactive systems for visual information processing

```
Y  A  H  Z  X  T
Z  H  B  C  T  M
N  F  A  P  Z  Y
K  L  Z  B  A  O
M  O  C  R  A  Z
A  S  Z  U  T  D
Q  B  P  Z  C  S
Z  C  M  T  L  O
H  Z  T  C  R  M
L  P  Z  T  W  B
Y  C  U  D  H  Z
G  Z  F  B  O  N
H  P  W  O  Z  S
Z  R  G  H  P  Q
O  X  A  Z  Y  D
F  Z  B  M  T  G
```

FIGURE 5.4 *Example of a test of visual search in which a target letter (Z) is to be detected under two conditions: clear and blurred print. Williams, Brannan, and Lartigue[32] used this visual search task and reported improved performance in subjects with reading dysfunction when the letters were slightly blurred.*

by suggesting that the transient system carries "global" visual information, whereas the sustained system transmits "detailed" visual information. This global-to-local mode of processing has been related to the M-cell/P-cell pathway, in which there appears to be a sequence to the flow of visual information.[53] It is possible that those with RD rely more heavily on "global" analysis than do normal readers, who are more analytic, or detail oriented, and use both global and local judgments in a visual search task. It seems reasonable to assume that, if there is a transient system deficit, interfering with the transmission of detailed visual information should enable the transient system to act in a more robust fashion to allow for transient-on-sustained inhibition, as suggested by Breitmeyer and Ganz.[10] The transient response precedes the sustained response, and output from the transient system affects the sustained response.

Williams, Brannan, and Lartigue[32] provided early evidence that the relationship between the two subsystems (transient and sustained) could be modified by reducing the impact of high spatial frequencies associated with the edges of letters and transmitted by the sustained subsystem. Williams, Lecluyse, and Rock-Faucheux[33] used red and blue filters, clear acetate for image blurring (as did Williams, Brannan, and Lartigue[32]), and modification of edge contrast by using dark or light gray backgrounds. Their subjects were children, 8–12 years old, with normal intelligence, color vision, visual acuity, auditory discrimination, and language ability. The children with RD were an average of 2.2 years delayed in their reading ability and were matched with the normal controls for age and intelligence.

The testing yielded a number of interesting results. First, use of the acetate filter improved the reading ability of the children with RD, thus confirming an earlier study.[32] Second, the blue filter yielded the same results as the neutral acetate filter, but the red filter did not. Third, the light gray background produced significant improvement in the reading comprehension of the poor readers compared to the white background. These three significant findings can be explained by assuming that the blue (short-wavelength) stimuli increase the transient systems processing rate in RD children and have essentially the same effect as blurring the text with the acetate filter. The use of the gray background, however, reduces the contrast of the letter edges, which has a negative effect on the sustained system, essentially reducing its impact on the transient system.

Tinted or Attenuating Filters

These conclusions lead to the possibility that there may be two ways to modify transient-on-sustained inhibition in people with RD. First, using blue filters, the weak transient system can be stimulated to produce a better transient-on-sustained response. Second, by using either the neutral acetate filter (blurring the image) or a gray background, the sustained system can be weakened, allowing the transient-on-sustained interaction to improve. Contrast reduction appears to be the key for establishing better reading performance in some individuals with RD. (See Chapter 12, Case Studies, for further discussion of dyslexia and tinted lenses.)

Irlen[54] promoted the use of colored filters to aid individuals with RD. Controversy exists about whether any kind of filter really does help individuals with RD to read more efficiently.[55-59] The issue is especially pertinent in cases of dyslexia. Dudeck et al.[60] found no significant correlation between dyseidesia and a magnocellular pathway defect in a sample of dyseidetic adults matched with normal readers who were not dyslexic when tested on contrast sensitivity functions with various sine wave gratings drifting at 1 and 10 Hz and also with visual-evoked potential testing. Borsting et al.[61-64] did find, however, a relation between a magnocellular pathway defect and dysphoneidesia in similar studies of adults. Further research is needed to determine the possible relations between magnocellular defects and the several types of dyslexia and whether severity of each type is a factor. Clinical implications of these issues are discussed in Part IV.

Summary

Controlling for intelligence, educational opportunity, and cultural differences, research suggests that, in a subpopulation of poor readers, there exists a low-level visual processing deficit. This deficit appears to occur early in the preattentive area in cortical processing of visual information, and is of sensory rather than maturational origin. The deficit appears to affect the transient aspects of visual information rather than the spatial and is expressed whenever there is a temporal component in the incoming visual information. The differences between normal readers and those with RD with transient visual system defects might be reduced or eliminated by visual conditions that reduce the impact of the high spatial frequency components in the visual information stream.

References

1. Bryant ND. Characteristics of dyslexia and their remedial implication. Except Child 1964;31:195–9.
2. Clifton-Everest IM. Dyslexia: is there a disorder of visual perception? Neuropsychologia 1976;14:491–4.
3. Vellutino FR, Pruzek RM, Steger JA, et al. Immediate visual recall in poor and normal readers as a function of age and orthographic-linguistic familiarity. Cortex 1973;9:370–86.
4. Vellutino FR, Steger JA, Kaman M, et al. Visual form perception in deficient and normal readers as a function of age and orthographic-linguistic familiarity. Cortex 1975;11:22–30.
5. Vellutino FR, Steger JA, Harding CJ, et al. Verbal vs. non-verbal paired-associates learning in poor and normal readers. Neuropsychologia 1975;13:75–82.
6. Fisher DF, Frankfurter A. Normal and disabled readers can locate and identify letters: where's the perceptual deficit? J Read Behav 1977;10:31–43.
7. Morrison FJ, Giordani B, Nagy J. Reading disability: an information-processing analysis. Science 1977;196:77–9.
8. Arnett JL, Di Lollo V. Visual information processing in relation to age and to reading ability. J Exp Child Psychol 1979;27:143–52.
9. Hulme C. The implausibility of low-level visual deficits as a cause of children's reading difficulty. Neurophysiology 1988;5:369–74.
10. Breitmeyer BG, Ganz L. Implications of sustained and transient channels for theories of visual pattern masking, saccadic suppression, and information processing. Psychol Rev 1976;83:1–36.
11. Stanley G, Hall R. Short-term visual information processing in dyslexics. Child Dev 1973;44:841–4.
12. Stanley G, Hall R. A comparison of dyslexics and normals in recalling letter arrays after brief presentation. Br J Educ Psychol 1973;43:301–4.
13. Stanley G. Visual Memory Processes in Dyslexia. In D Deutsch, JA Deutsch (eds), Short-Term Memory. New York: Academic, 1975;182–94.
14. Lovegrove W, Brown C. Development of information processing in normal and disabled readers. Percept Mot Skills 1978;46:1047–54.
15. Lyle JG, Goyen JD. Effect of speed of exposure and difficulty of discrimination on visual recognition of retarded readers. J Abnorm Psychol 1975;84:673–6.

16. Lyle JG, Goyen JD. Visual recognition, developmental lag and strephosymbolia in reading retardation. J Abnorm Psychol 1968;73:25–9.
17. Lovegrove W, Billing G, Slaghuis W. Processing of visual contour orientation information in normal and disabled reading children. Cortex 1978;14:268–78.
18. Lovegrove WJ, Heddle M, Slaghuis W. Reading disability: spatial frequency deficits in visual information store. Neuropsychologia 1980;18:111–5.
19. Badcock D, Lovegrove W. The effects of contrast, stimulus duration, and spatial frequency on visible persistence in normal and specifically disabled readers. J Exp Psychol Hum Percept Perform 1981;7:495–505.
20. Lovegrove W, Martin F, Slaghuis W. A theoretical and experimental case for a visual deficit in specific reading disability. Cogn Neuropsychol 1986;3:225–67.
21. Lovegrove WJ, Bowling A, Badcock D, et al. Specific reading disability: differences in contrast sensitivity as a function of spatial frequency. Science 1980;210:439–40.
22. Slaghuis WL, Lovegrove W. Flicker masking of spatial frequency dependent visible persistence and specific reading disability. Perception 1984;13:527–34.
23. Breitmeyer BG, Levi DM, Harwerth RS. Flicker masking in spatial vision. Vision Res 1981;21:1377–85.
24. Martin F, Lovegrove W. The effects of field size and luminance on contrast sensitivity differences between specifically reading disabled and normal children. Neuropsychologia 1984;22:73–7.
25. Martin F, Lovegrove W. Flicker contrast sensitivity in normal and specifically disabled readers. Perception 1987;16:215–21.
26. Brannan JR, Williams MC. The effects of age and reading ability on flicker threshold. Clin Vis Sci 1988;3:137–42.
27. Martin F, Lovegrove WJ. Uniform-field flicker masking in control and specifically-disabled readers. Perception 1988;17:203–14.
28. Williams MC, Bologna NB. Perceptual grouping effects in good and poor readers. Percept Psychophys 1985;38:367–74.
29. May JG, Williams MC, Dunlop WP. Temporal order judgments in good and poor readers. Neuropsychologia 1988;26:917–24.
30. Brannan JR, Williams MC. Allocation of visual attention in good and poor readers. Percept Psychophys 1987;41:23–8.
31. Brannan JR, Williams MC. Developmental versus sensory deficit effects on perceptual processing in the reading disabled. Percept Psychophys 1988;44:437–44.
32. Williams MC, Brannan JR, Lartigue EK. Visual search in good and poor readers. Clin Vis Sci 1987;1:367–71.
33. Williams MC, Lecluyse K, Rock-Faucheux A. Effective interventions for reading disability. J Am Optom Assoc 1992;63:411–7.
34. Gibson EJ. Learning to read. Science 1965;148:1066–72.
35. Gibson JJ, Radner M. Adaptation, aftereffect and contrast in the perception of tilted lines. I. Quantitative studies. J Exp Psychol Gen 1937;20:453–67.
36. Bodis-Wollner I. Visual acuity and contrast sensitivity in patients with cerebral lesions. Science 1972;178:769–71.
37. Bodis-Wollner I, Hendley C. On the separability of two mechanisms involved in the detection of grating patterns in humans. J Physiol (Lond) 1985;291:251–63.

38. Bowling A. The effects of peripheral movement and flicker on the detection thresholds of sinusoidal gratings. Percept Psychophys 1985;37:181–8.
39. Pantle AJ. Temporal determinants of spatial sine-wave masking. Vision Res 1983;23:749–57.
40. Bowling A, Lovegrove W. The effect of stimulus duration on the persistence of gratings. Percept Psychophys 1980;27:574–8.
41. Bowling A, Lovegrove W. Response times to different spatial frequencies. Is there a 100-msec rule? Percept Psychophys 1980;28:599–600.
42. Fletcher JM, Satz P. Unitary deficit hypotheses of reading disabilities: has Vellutino led us astray? J Learn Disabil 1979;12:155–9.
43. Navon D. Forest before trees: the precedence of global features in visual perception. Cogn Psychol 1977;9:353–83.
44. Breitmeyer BG. Unmasking visual masking: a look at the "why" behind the veil of the "how." Psychol Rev 1980;87:52–69.
45. Vienet JC., Duvernoy J, Tribillon G, et al. Three methods of information assessment for optical data processing. Appl Optom 1973;12:950–60.
46. Di Lollo V. Temporal characteristics of iconic memory. Nature 1977;267:241–3.
47. Di Lollo V, Wilson AE. Iconic persistence and perceptual moment as determinants of temporal integration in vision. Vision Res 1978;18:1607–10.
48. Lovegrove WJ, Meyer GE. Visible persistence as a function of spatial frequency, number of cycles and retinal area. Vision Res 1984;24:255–9.
49. Dzn H De Lange. Research into the dynamic nature of the human fovea-cortex systems with intermittent and modulated light. I. Attenuation characteristics with white and colored light. J Opt Soc Am 1958;48:777–84.
50. Pomerantz JR, Gardner WR. Stimulus configuration in selective attention tasks. Percept Psychophys 1973;14:565–9.
51. Pomerantz JR, Schwaitzberg SD. Grouping by proximity: selective attention measures. Percept Psychophys 1975;18:355–61.
52. Williams MC, Weisstein N. Perceptual grouping produces spatial-frequency specific effects on metacontrast (abstract). Invest Ophthalmol Vis Sci 1980;19(suppl):165.
53. Bassi CJ, Lehmkuhle S. Clinical implications of parallel visual pathways. J Am Optom Assoc 1990;61:98–110.
54. Irlen H. Successful treatment of learning disabilities. Presentation at the 91st annual meeting of the American Psychological Association, 1983.
55. Scheiman M, Blaskey P, Ciner EB, et al. Vision characteristics of individuals identified as Irlen Filter candidates. J Am Optom Assoc 1990;61:600–5.
56. Evans BJW, Drasdo N. Tinted lenses and related therapies for learning disabilities: a review. Ophthalmic Physiol Opt 1991;11:206–17.
57. Menacker SJ, Breton ME, Breton ML, et al. Do tinted lenses improve the performance of dyslexic children? A cohort study. Arch Ophthalmol 1993;111:213–8.
58. Cardinal DN, Griffin JR, Christenson GN. Do tinted lenses really help students with reading disabilities? Intervention School Clin 1993;28:275–9.
59. Scheiman M. Scotopic sensitivity syndrome, reading disability and vision disorders. J Behav Optom 1994;5;63–6.

60. Dudeck K, Kelley C, Borsting E, et al. Contrast sensitivity functions in the dyseidetic dyslexic. Research paper on file in the M.B. Ketchum Memorial Library of the Southern California College of Optometry, Fullerton, CA, 1993.
61. Borsting E, Ridder WH III. Does the dysphoneidetic dyslexic have a magnocellular defect? Presented at the annual meeting of the American Academy of Optometry, San Diego, CA, Dec. 13, 1994.
62. Ridder WH III, Borsting E. Which dyslexic subtypes demonstrate a magnocellular pathway defect? Presented at the annual meeting of the American Academy of Optometry, San Diego, CA, Dec. 13, 1994.
63. Borsting E, Ridder WH III, Dudeck K, et al. The presence of a magnocellular defect depends on the type of dyslexia. Vision Res 1995;36:1047–53.
64. Ridder WH III, Borsting E, Cooper M, et al. Not all dyslexics are created equal. Invest Ophthalmol Vis Sci 1995;36(suppl):673.

6

Development of Higher-Order Visual Skills for Information Processing

The development of vision affects the process of learning to read. Components of vision discussed here include vision efficiency, visual-perceptual skills, and visual-motor skills. Details of the developmental process provide background information on specifics of these skills in relation to academic achievement. Multivariate analysis of these skills is related to reading achievement in general and then specifically to dyslexia.

This information forms a foundation for later presentations on methods of testing and management of visual deficiencies related to reading dysfunction (RD). The clinician can then conceptualize total management and how it may differ between nondyslexic and dyslexic RD.

Development of Vision and Its Impact on Learning to Read

Development of higher-order visual skills can be discussed in the context of learning. Learning occurs as a complex multilevel process involving sensation, perception, imagery, language, symbolization, and, finally, conceptualization.[1] If a link in the hierarchic chain from sensation to conceptualization is broken, the process of learning is impeded. Reduced visual acuity, for example, adversely affects visual perception; likewise, a visual perception problem adversely affects the development of symbolization and conceptualization.[2] A significant positive correlation between test results for visual-perceptual development and reading readiness has been found for children in kindergarten and the early primary grades.[3] This is in accord with the general notion that good perceptual-motor ability is a necessary component of reading readiness. Visual-perceptual development, therefore, is an important aspect to consider in the learning-to-read process of children in the early grades.

Vision development can be modeled as a multidimensional process involving (1) gathering light, (2) processing impulses, and (3) integrating visual impulses with other sensory impulses and the motor system. Problems in visual development can, therefore, adversely affect reading.

Gathering light involves anatomic and functional characteristics of the binocular system. Light must be accurately focused on the retina, the two eyes must fuse efficiently on the object of regard, and good oculomotor control of saccades and fixations is necessary for gathering visual information in the act of reading. A brief discussion of these skills leads to an understanding of visual tracking (oculomotor function), focusing (accommodation), eye teaming (vergence abilities), and how these aspects relate to the process of reading. Development of tracking, focusing, and teaming skills occurs rapidly during the first few months of life. Rudimentary abilities in these areas exist by 3–4 months of age.[4–6] These skills are further refined as they are applied to the more complex tasks required in school. (Developmentally appropriate testing procedures for vision efficiency skills are covered in Chapter 9.) Evaluation of visual skills efficiency (VSE) is an attempt to determine how clearly, comfortably, and quickly a patient can perform far and near tasks. Examples of behavioral signs and symptoms of poor vision efficiency are listed in Table 6.1. Unlike adults, children may not recognize these symptoms as abnormal and, therefore, they may simply avoid near tasks and become easily distracted.

TABLE 6.1   Behavioral Signs and Symptoms of Inefficient Visual Skills

Oculomotor dysfunction
    Skipping and rereading words
    Losing place while reading
    Using a finger as pointer
    Difficulty with copying tasks
Accommodative dysfunction
    Blurred vision when focusing from far to near
    Fluctuating clarity
    Rubbing eyes
    Asthenopia
Vergence dysfunction
    Double vision
    Blurring of print
    Print running together
    Asthenopia

Although we have segregated the areas of vision efficiency skills and perception, in practice they function in an integrated, synchronous, and inseparable fashion. School children are expected to have the ability to direct visual attention and maintain accurate focus and binocular alignment under a variety of conditions. They must be able to perform these synchronous actions accurately, effortlessly, and virtually automatically.[7]

Visual Skills Efficiency

Is RD related to poor VSE? Evidence supports the idea that eye movement problems are associated with reading and learning problems.[8–12] Oculomotor errors include an abnormal number of fixations, regressions, longer durations of fixation, and a shorter span of perception.[13–17] In spite of these correlative data, the primacy of eye movements in reading proficiency has been debated: Is RD due to poor eye movements, or is it caused by a primary cognitive problem? Research has addressed this question and demonstrated that many with RD do have oculomotor problems, even when the tracking material contains no written language component (e.g., rows of dots).[18, 19]

Unfortunately, there have been no well-documented studies addressing the issue of dyseidetic and dysphonetic subtypes as to the relation with oculomotor problems. Investigations have included both general RD and specific RD (dyslexia) and thus muddied the waters. We believe, from clinical experience, that poor oculomotor skills can result in general RD but that they do not cause specific RD. Poor oculomotor skills, however, probably contribute to the RD of an individual with dyslexia. This concept helps explain why many with dyslexia may have good oculomotor skills while many nondyslexics with eye movement problems may have general RD.

Accommodation (eye focusing) is another visual skill found to be a factor in reading ability. Difficulties with the accommodative system have been associated with symptoms such as blur at near and when changing fixation from near to far, a tendency to hold near work too close, frontal headaches as a result of extended near work, and asthenopia.[20] These factors often lead to great difficulty with school work and avoidance of reading. A number of investigators have reported high prevalences of accommodative dysfunction among children with RD and learning disabilities.[9–12, 21] Furthermore, a multivariate analysis determined that up to 8% of the variance in reading ability could be predicted by an individual's accommodative accuracy.[22]

The status of binocularity is also an important factor in the reading process. Accurate coordination of the two eyes is required for fusion and good stereopsis. Of great importance is the comfort and efficiency with which fusion is attained and maintained. Symptoms associated with poor binocularity include asthenopia, double vision, words running together, pulling or drawing sensations, and frontal headaches.[23–25] If no symptoms are found in cases of binocular dysfunction, the patient may be suppressing an eye[26] or avoiding near tasks.[27] We have seen many patients with binocular problems who cover an eye to avoid symptoms, particularly with prolonged reading tasks.

The prevalence of binocular anomalies has been reported to be higher than normal among populations of learning disabled individuals.[9–12, 28–33] Furthermore, binocular fusion skills can be used to separate poor from normal readers.[34, 35] Robust data support the theory that binocular anomalies can contribute to RD. Because of symptoms that impede the act of visually gathering information, the task of reading is more difficult.

Reviews of the literature by Simons and Grisham[36] and meta-analysis of past studies by Simons and Gassler[37] have shed some light on this important issue. The binocular variables of exophoria at near, vertical phoria, fusional reserves, convergence insufficiency, and fixation disparity are associated with below-average reading performance. As to refractive status, adverse factors are hyperopia, anisometropia, and aniseikonia; myopia, however, is associated with average and above-average reading performance. Evans et al.[38] found that binocular anomalies are not the cause of specific RD, but are likely to make most reading tasks more of a burden. Therefore, those deficiencies and their associated symptoms should be managed with lenses, prisms, vision training, or a combination of these tools.

Does strabismus cause reading difficulty? It is known that a severe dysfunction of fusional ability may cause a person to experience a loss of sensory fusion (suppression). This may lead to strabismus. Eames,[32] Cassin,[39] and Hoffman[9] presented evidence of a slightly higher prevalence of strabismus in learning disabled children, but other research does not demonstrate that strabismus is a major determinant of RD. It stands to reason, however, that an intermittent eye-turn with associated diplopia and possible visual confusion would interfere with reading efficiency. On the other hand, a case of constant strabismus with deep suppression would eliminate the confusion and diplopia and, therefore, not necessarily be a problem with regard to visual demands of reading. The reason a higher prevalence of learning disability is found in the strabismic population may be due to the higher prevalence of strabismus in neurologically handicapped individuals (e.g., those with Down syndrome). In developmentally normal individuals, however, we do not believe strabismus that is constant and unilateral is a highly significant adverse factor in reading and scholarly achievement.

Visual-Perceptual-Motor Development

Visual-perceptual-motor (VPM) development is a learned, dynamic process.[40] The eye does not simply provide an exact duplication of the physical world. Rather, what is eventually "seen" requires selective attention, comparison with past events, and integration with other senses. The act of visually perceiving involves more than simply that which is visible. An understanding of the visual-developmental process is embodied in the analogy of the conditioned and unconditioned reflexes described by Lyle.[41] For example, a newborn foal comes into the world equipped with the visual and motor functions necessary to gallop away from danger. The ability to discriminate visually and guide motor movements only a short time after birth is apparently due to an inborn unconditioned reflex. This visual-perceptual apparatus in the horse is complete at birth and virtually ready to respond before it is actually put to use.

In contrast, the human infant is completely dependent on another human being for its existence. In its first few days, an infant's behavior is much the same whether or not the eyes are open. The child is unable to orient itself with respect to gravity or visual space. Ocular movements are initially of a wandering, aimless variety. "They are not, however, uncoordinated movements, but rather co-coordinated movements of version and vergence, although at first rarely related to any specific object stimulus. Later, further coordination of the movements develops with reference to the stimulus of visible objects."[41] Without proper sensorimotor stimulation, VPM development may be severely hampered or incompletely acquired.[42, 43] Furthermore, it has been demonstrated in cats (and, therefore, theoretically in humans) that physiologic maladaptations resulting from deprived sensorimotor experience may be reversed with proper intervention.[44, 45] In this context a discussion of VPM development in children is relevant.

Suchoff[46] pointed out the nature of visual development from infancy through early childhood. He made the distinction between the reflex-like action of visual attentiveness in the infant versus more purposeful use of vision during later infancy and early childhood. His theory of visual-spatial development, based on the cognitive developmental scheme of Piaget, presents an empiric appreciation of the relation between visual development and reading and the importance of sub-skills of visual perception to reading.

Barsch[47] alluded to the fact that, with regard to body orientation, "front" space is developed first in the infant, progressing to "side" space, which is developed later in childhood. "Down" space is tentatively organized early in life, with "up" space being refined later, and "back" space developing last. Gesell et al. also describe spatial development as a process wherein the child unites discrete spatial areas over the years from infancy into childhood. During this process the discrete areas are eventually unified into a continuous whole.[48]

The process of visual-spatial development may be understood by considering an overview of the child's changing ability to manipulate visual space cognitively throughout the early years. Before the age of 2.5 years, the child operates primarily in near space. After this age, areas beyond arm's length increasingly begin to attract the child's attention, although there is difficulty shifting attention back and forth between near and far. Age 3.5 is a transitional time that is necessary to arrive at some integrated spatial sense, which begins at about age 5. At age 6, awareness emerges of objects and their positions in space, both relative to other objects and to the child. For the 8-year-old, a new distinction is made with the realization that a person viewing an object from a different location can have a different perspective. The child begins to appreciate the concept of multiple perspectives. During these years, the child has progressed from a stimulus-bound, reflex-dominated, visual style to a mastery level of viewing, organizing, and cognitively manipulating his or her visual space.

Having presented general visual-spatial development, we can move on to specific visual-perceptual abilities acquired in the developmental process. This leads to a rationale for evaluation of specific subskills of VPM development in the child. As mentioned earlier, Suchoff[46] applied the piagetian framework of cognitive development to a scheme for acquisition of visual-perceptual skills. Piaget and Inhelder[49] regarded visual-spatial development as a subdivision of intellectual development. Therefore, we present Piaget's model of the periods and subperiods of cognitive development. The four main periods are (1) *sensorimotor* (birth to 2 years), (2) *preoperations* (2–7 years), (3) *concrete operations* (7–11 years), and (4) *formal operations* (11 years and older). By relating the areas of cognitive and visual development, certain principles become evident. The process of visual development is a hierarchy proceeding from a tactual approach in infancy to a predominantly visual approach in later childhood (this was Kephart's approach, later espoused by Getman[50]). In between, the intermediate stages of tactual-visual and then visual-tactual strategies arise. These can be viewed as interwoven with the stages of Piaget's model. Getman's hypothesis[50] was that "vision develops under the tutelage of touch."

The sensorimotor period involves the child's ability to act on physical objects directly in the physical present. In general, the child lacks the symbolic and representational ability to conceptualize in the absence of physical stimuli. At this stage, the child also does not know whether the apparent change of the shape of an object is a result of his or her own movement or movement of the object. As a result, the child often perceives an object whose orientation has been changed as a completely different object (e.g., a chair turned upside down). This stage begins in infancy, when visual behavior is initially guided by innate reflexes (e.g., tonic neck reflex), and ends with the 2-year-old being able to combine pertinent information from all senses and understand that this sensory information is from a single object. For example, a child bouncing a rubber ball is aware of its sight, sound, and touch sensations and can relate these sensations to the rubber ball. The child also understands cause and effect and may begin to plan visual-motor activities.

In the preoperations period the child gradually begins to acquire representational thought, or the ability to conceptualize people and objects even though they are not physically present. Language is a key factor in this development because words are used to represent objects that are not present. Also during this stage, the child begins to understand visual space in terms of its multiple dimensions. Looking out the window of an airplane, a child at this stage would not say "Look at the toy cars below" but instead, "We must be a long way from the cars because they look so small." This representational ability is taken a step further and applied to physical manipulations that require logical consideration of two aspects of visual information. For example, a preoperational child, when faced with a glass of water poured from a short, wide container into a tall, narrow container would say incorrectly that there is now more water than there was in the first container.

The ability to use representational reasoning applied to higher-level tasks in the concrete operations period is a tenet of Piaget's theory. He contended that there is an upward spiraling of development. Behavioral patterns are continually repeated until they are mastered, at which time they may then be applied to more complex situations. The last period, usually age 11 or older, formal operations, is notable for the child's ability to deal with abstract principles and theories by freeing himself or herself to an even greater degree from the physical present.

Visual-Spatial Organization

Suchoff[46] described a second major component of visual development involving an important aspect of vision in humans: the organization and manipulation of visual space (as in the development of directionality from laterality). The individual must learn how to reference objects in space. For the infant who has not begun to accomplish this task, the world is a very disordered and confusing realm that must continually be explored tactually to attempt to establish some semblance of order. First, the individual must establish a reference point, or an origin, from which to make spatial judgments. The common reference point is the self because objects are localized with regard to the observer. This reference point has been referred to as the *invariant*, meaning that one's body becomes the reference point from which structure and order develop.[46, 51] The body becomes the origin from which objects in the environment are perceived as being left, right, up, down, front, back, or larger and smaller. Therefore, the organization and awareness of the self (the invariant) must occur before the individual can organize spatial aspects of vision.

The notion of making directional judgments in space involves the process of lateralization, which occurs during childhood. This concept is best appreciated based on comments by Early:[52] "The child develops an internal awareness of left and right from his internal awareness that the body has two sides. The inner awareness is called laterality, which becomes part of the motor base. Space is organized as the child receives information from the world and matches it to his internally organized motor base." Barsch[47] held that this process begins when the infant experiences himself or herself as a two-sided individual as a result of the tonic neck reflex (in which the head is turned to one side and the hand on that side of the body is reflexively extended). In this way, the child may begin to explore aspects of his or her two-sidedness. The process continues as various crawling and creeping patterns develop. Similar patterns are repeated as the child begins walking. An overview of normal child development is given by Cron.[53]

Cratty[54] described four stages in the acquisition of right-left awareness:

1. The child is unable to distinguish between the two sides of his or her body from birth to about age 3.5 years.
2. The child becomes aware that his or her left and right limbs are found on either side of the body but is unaware of which body parts are *called* left and right (age 4–5 years).
3. The child realizes that symmetric left and right body parts are found on opposite sides of the body (age 6–7 years).
4. The child can precisely identify which parts of the body are right and left (age 8–9 years).

TABLE 6.2   Categories of Visual-Perceptual-Motor (VPM) Evaluation*

Bilateral integration, laterality, and directionality
Motor-free visual perception (e.g., visual discrimination, form perception, visual memory, and visualization)
Visual-motor integration
Auditory-visual integration (customarily included in VPM assessment)

*VPM evaluation is also known clinically as *visual information–processing evaluation.*
Source: Modified from LG Hoffman, MW Rouse. Referral recommendations for binocular function and/or developmental perceptual deficiencies. J Am Optom Assoc 1980;51:119–25.

Piaget,[55] however, contended that children are able to distinguish their own right and left sides by age 6. Benton[56] was in general agreement with Piaget as to the age of right-left awareness.

The next area of discussion is VPM development in children. The issue is to determine what, if any, relation exists between VPM development and early achievement in school. It will be demonstrated that VPM skills are necessary for the child to begin to deal with visual symbols used to convey meaning (e.g., numbers, letters, words).

Assessment of VPM skills can be categorized into four broad areas[20] (Table 6.2). Motor-free visual perception can be further divided in several subareas. A test often used for VPM skills assessment is the Test for Visual Perceptual Skills (TVPS).[57] This test includes assessment of visual discrimination, visual form constancy, visual figure-ground, visual memory, visual spatial relations, visual sequential memory, and visual closure. These skills are acquired as part of the developmental process.

This brief overview of Piaget's theory and the role of lateralization sets the stage for a discussion of the relation between VPM development and (1) early school achievement, (2) reading, and (3) dyslexia.

Visual-Perceptual-Motor Development and Early Achievement in School

VPM development (also referred to as development of *visual information processing*) has several components. Each component is related to academic readiness and achievement. A strong correlation between VPM development and learning is evidenced by multivariate analysis, which considers all components of VPM development. These data are presented after a brief discussion of the individual components of VPM development and their role in learning.

One purpose of the VPM system is to filter out extraneous stimuli, so that meaning can be extracted from the environment by processing only the pertinent stimuli.[58] The resulting organized perceptions allow for stability, order, and predictability in the individual's ability to deal with environmental demands. A deficit in VPM development causes the child to have difficulty organizing his or her perceptual world, which leads to a sense of being lost among the vast array of competing stimuli. Coleman[59] stated that, "If a child perceives his space world with confusion and distortion, academic learning will probably be difficult no matter what the measured level of intelligence." Four categories of VPM development are discussed: (1) bilateral integration, laterality, and directionality; (2) visual discrimination and form perception; (3) visual memory and visualization; and (4) visual-motor integration. (Auditory perception and auditory-visual integration are discussed in Chapters 8, 9, and 11.)

Bilateral Integration, Laterality, and Directionality

The ability of the individual to guide the motor system visually while maintaining awareness of body parts on both sides is critical for efficient use of visual space.[60] This is the VPM component of bilateral integration; it depends on the *invariant*, as described earlier. Movement of the body is the foundation for virtually all behavior.[61] The invariant in academic performance appears to be related to the area of selective attention. Three aspects of attention have been identified by Keogh: (1) coming to attention, (2) decision making, and (3) sustaining attention over time.[62] According to Keogh, the skills for coming to attention and controlling attention are influenced by the individual's ability to use motor activity appropriately. Therefore, the invariant appears to be an important factor for selective attention. Bilateral integration is also a requisite for development of laterality and directionality. The invariant must develop as a stable frame of reference to ensure good right and left discrimination.

The internal awareness of the left and right sides of the body is termed *laterality*. The projection of this awareness into space allows for consistent directional judgments, as in the ability to differentiate between the letters *b* and *d*. This skill, called *directionality*, is critical for recognition of letters in the early stages of learning to read.[63] This is supported by the finding that letter reversal problems occur in association with delayed development of laterality and directionality.[64–66] Furthermore, Kaufman[67] reported that correlations between letter reversals and poor reading achievement were statistically significant.

Visual Discrimination and Form Perception

The abilities to recognize a specific form and to differentiate between unlike forms are the perceptual skills of *visual discrimination* and *visu-*

al form perception. Theories of perception dictate an initial step involving discrimination,[63, 68, 69] but visual discrimination and form perception are difficult to separate clinically. These skills also require the individual to be able to (1) synthesize various components of visual stimuli into a single percept, (2) identify visual forms with reduced clues (i.e., closure), and (3) recognize forms embedded in complex irrelevant patterns (i.e., figure-ground).[58]

Barrett[70] emphasized that visual discrimination is a widely accepted measure of reading readiness. Support for this contention has been provided by a number of investigators.[71-75] Visual figure-ground deficiencies are prevalent in children with learning disabilities and have been highly correlated with poor attention.[76] Additionally, research has demonstrated that deficient form perception is common among children with reading problems.[77-80] Even among proponents of language dysfunctions in reading difficulties, emphasis is placed on visual readiness skills for reading.[81]

Visual Memory and Visualization

The perceptual functions of visual memory and visualization are closely related. Visual memory is the foundation for visualization and involves the ability to store and recall visually presented information.

Visual memory is important for academic achievement, and deficiencies in this area have been reported with a prevalence of 72–80% in learning-disabled populations.[9, 12] Deficits in the following areas related to visual memory have also been associated with RD: (1) temporal order perception,[82] (2) short-term memory,[83] (3) visual-spatial order perception,[84] and (4) visual information processing.[85]

Visualization involves the use of stored and recalled information in a mentally manipulative way so that multiple perspectives can be appreciated. This ability facilitates all learning.[82] Many vision testing and training procedures involve visualization.

Visual-Motor Integration

Visual-motor integration (VMI) has been characterized as a complicated integrative function that involves both visual perception and purposeful motoric action as a means of acting on the perception.[86, 87] In this process, the individual must integrate the visual-perceptual and fine motor systems. For example, paper and pencil tasks require good VMI skills.[11] VMI deficiencies have been found prevalent (92%) in the learning-disabled population.[9, 12, 88] There have also been correlative studies relating VMI deficiencies to RD[9, 12, 87-92] and other support for the predictive value of visual-motor tests for future reading achievement.[93-100] Development of VMI serves as a foundation for spatial orientation, symbol identification, and, eventually, for reading achievement.

Multivariate Analysis of Visual-Perceptual-Motor Skills and Reading Achievement

VPM development has been elucidated by explaining (1) the associated developmental process, (2) its component skill areas, and (3) the relation of the components to academic areas. To appreciate the impact of VPM development on reading, one must consider the additive nature of visual-perceptual skills. This concept was carefully investigated by Solan and Mozlin[3] in a multiple regression analysis that correlated test results involving visual discrimination, form perception, fine motor control, auditory-visual integration, and visual memory to reading readiness and reading achievement in the early grades. The results of this analysis demonstrated the robust relation between reading readiness in kindergarten, reading achievement in the first grade, and VPM skills. Statistical variance of more than 50% was shown, but predictability was not high. The investigators also found that the strength of the correlation in multivariate analysis decreased by the end of the second grade. They offered the explanation that, as the child matures, the role of language acquisition and cognitive considerations take on primacy in the development of reading ability. Nevertheless, they showed the critical role of VPM development as a part of the process of reading acquisition.

Relation Between Visual-Perceptual-Motor Development and Dyslexia

With an understanding of VPM development and its role in reading, the relation between VPM development and dyslexia is considered. Vellutino[101] underscored the confusion regarding visual perception and dyslexia. His contention was that dyslexia is not correctable by means of therapies designed to "strengthen" the visual-spatial system. In effect, he argued that dyslexia was not a primary result of visual deficits. He felt that dyslexia is a dysfunction of storage and retrieval of linguistic information rather than a consequence of a defect in the visual system. How can this notion be reconciled with previous findings on the connection between VPM development and reading? To address this issue Griffin and Borghi conducted a clinical study (unpublished) using the model of types of dyslexia presented in Chapter 3 to investigate the correlation between VPM skills and specific types of dyslexia. The purpose was to determine what, if any, relation existed between dyseidetic and dysphonetic dyslexia and various VPM test results, which included the Birch-Belmont Auditory-Visual Integration Test (BB), Motor-Free Visual Perception Test (MVPT), Jordan Left-Right Reversal Test (JLRRT), and the Beery Developmental Test of VMI (BVMI). Subjects included 22 children (four females, 18 males)

TABLE 6.3   Perceptual Test Scores in Study of Comparison with Dyslexia

Rank	Perceptual Age Equivalent
1 (very weak)	2 or more years < chronologic age
2 (weak)	1–2 years < chronologic age
3 (adequate)	±1 year of chronologic age
4 (strong)	1–2 years > chronologic age
5 (very strong)	2 or more years > chronologic age

Source: Unpublished study at The Southern California College of Optometry (JR Griffin and R Borghi).

TABLE 6.4   Dyslexia Determination Test Encoding Results

Rank	Dyseidetic or Dysphonetic Encoding
1 (very weak)	<20%
2 (weak)	20–39%
3 (adequate)	40–59%
4 (strong)	60–79%
5 (very strong)	80–100%

Source: Unpublished study at The Southern California College of Optometry (JR Griffin and R Borghi).

TABLE 6.5   Correlation Coefficient (r) Matrix Comparing Visual-Perceptual-Motor Results with Dyslexia Results (Tables 6.3 and 6.4)

	Dysphonesia	Dyseidesia	JLRRT	MVPT	BVMI
Dyseidesia	−0.456	—	—	—	—
JLRRT	−0.213	0.142	—	—	—
MVPT	−0.059	0.282	0.503	—	—
BVMI	−0.304	0.439	0.397	0.545	—
BB	0.494	−0.405	0.027	0.253	0.226

JLRRT = Jordan Left-Right Reversal Test; MVPT = Motor-Free Visual-Perception Test; BVMI = Beery Developmental Test of Visual-Motor Integration; BB = Birch-Belmont Auditory-Visual Integration Test.
Source: Unpublished study at The Southern California College of Optometry (JR Griffin and R Borghi).

referred to the Optometric Center of Fullerton, Vision Therapy Clinic, of the Southern California College of Optometry by teachers who noted that these children had difficulties in reading and academic performance. Subjects ranged in age from 7 to 9 years. Children were ranked from 1–5 for statistical analysis. Table 6.3 shows perceptual test results and Table 6.4 shows dyslexia test scores.

Pearson correlation coefficients are shown in Table 6.5 and are based on dyslexia rankings versus visual-perceptual rankings (JLRRT, MVPT, BB, and BVMI). We found that correlations between dyslexia and perceptual rankings were too weak to provide statistical significance. Positive clinical trends, however, were found between dysphonesia and the BB (r 0.494), and dyseidesia and the BVMI (r 0.439). Negative clinical trends (as would be expected) were shown between dysphonesia and the BVMI, and between dyseidesia and the BB.

Griffin et al.[102] investigated the relation between dyseidetic dyslexia, as diagnosed with the Dyslexia Determination Test (DDT),[103] and visual perception, as assessed with TVPS.[57] The sample included 30 subjects (aged 6–13 years). Categories of DDT results ranged from no dyslexia to increasing severities of dyseidetic dyslexia. The TVPS subtests included visual discrimination, visual memory, visual-spatial relations, visual form constancy, visual sequential memory, visual figure-ground, and visual closure. TVPS results were also ranked according to severity: (1) very weak (>1 year below chronologic age), (2) weak (7 months–1 year below chronologic age), (3) adequate (±6 months of chronologic age), (4) strong (7 months–1 year above chronologic age), (5) very strong (>1 year above chronologic age). Both multivariate and univariate analysis of variance indicated no statistical differences and no trends of clinical significance. These results are consistent with our contention that reading problems due to dyslexia (dyseidetic dyslexia in this study) and reading problems due to visual-perceptual deficiencies are of different etiologies. The same conclusion was reached in a similar study comparing dysphonetic dyslexia (DDT and TVPS results).[104] Although the previous two correlation studies found no relation between either dyseidetic or dysphonetic dyslexia and TVPS results, we believe visual-perceptual dysfunctions are adverse factors in the development of reading skills, especially in kindergarten and the first two grades.

Solan and Ficarra[105] discussed the differences between spatial-simultaneous and verbal-successive skills required in reading, which could be an explanation for the low correlation between the DDT and the TVPS. (Spatial-simultaneous processing is presumably tested with the TVPS, whereas verbal-successive skills are presumably tested with the DDT.)

Solan and Groffman[106] elaborated on this dichotomy by stating that, "Normally achieving children in kindergarten and grade 1 more often employed simultaneous processing for form and word recognition, but by the end of grade 2, . . . verbal-successive (sequential) skills . . . predominate." We interpret their conclusion as implying that a child in kindergarten or first grade would naturally try to decode words on a look-say (eidetic) basis, as in the formerly used "Dick and Jane" books (e.g., "Run, run, run, Spot. See Spot run."). This whole-word approach is eidetic decoding as opposed to phonetic (word-attack) decoding that is taught (or should be taught) in the first and second grades; phonetic decoding requires verbal-successive skills. Later on, however, the child again begins to rely progressively more on eidetic decoding because it is much more efficient than phonetic decoding. Solan and Groffman[106] reported that the variances for sucessive and simultaneous processing with reading were equal in a sample of normally achieving readers in grades 4 and 5. We believe they are implying that a *simultaneous processing dysfunction* would result in *dyseidesia* (which would be handicapping to a kindergartner or first-grader trying to recognize whole words on an eidetic decoding basis). Similarly, a first-grader with a *verbal-successive dysfunction* would have *dysphonesia* (and have word-attack trouble when trying to decode on a phonetic basis).

Groffman[107] links dyseidetic dyslexia to low simultaneous processing and dysphonetic dyslexia with low successive processing. He defines simultaneous processing as "the interpretation of separate elements into a whole . . . in a holistic fashion with a gestalt-like integration of information." Groffman's analogy is "locating the Big Dipper in the night sky." A clinical test would be one for visual figure-ground skill (see Chapter 9). On the other hand, successive (sequential) processing "involves information arriving in the brain in a serial order." Groffman's analogy is "counting the number of stars in the Big Dipper." A clinical test would be the visual sequential memory subtest of the TVPS (see Chapter 9). Although it is intriguing to think that visual-perceptual testing can detect and diagnose dyslexia on the basis of the simultaneous-successive dichotomy, this could, at best, be only an *indirect* method for dyslexia testing. Direct testing (see Chapter 10) is necessary for ruling dyslexia in or out in a patient with RD. There may be negligence if the optometrist fails to do so and management of the case is mishandled. Although the correlations are not high between VPM results and dyseidetic or dysphonetic dyslexia,[102–104] visual-perception evaluation is important and necessary in cases of RD. This is also particularly pertinent in cases of dysnemkinesia (see Chapter 10). Poor readers tend to reverse letters while reading and writing, and Groffman discussed several theories of the cause of these reversals,[107] but he recommended vision-perception therapy in appropriate cases (see Chapter 11).

We believe that visual-perceptual deficits cannot be conclusively equated with dyslexia. This is in accord with Vellutino.[101] This does not mean that VPM development is unimportant for reading and academic achievement. We have presented data demonstrating that VSE and VPM deficits can contribute to a dyslexic individual's overall difficulty in reading and learning. Even though these deficits probably do not cause dyslexia, a nondyslexic individual may have a general RD due to VSE or VPM problems, or both. Therefore, the importance of VSE and VPM development cannot be negated in reading problems by using the rationalization that "they do not cause dyslexia." These visual functions are of vital importance in the overall assessment and management of individuals with RD. Furthermore, this knowledge supports the rationale that vision therapy is a valid and viable treatment option in cases of learning difficulties, particularly RD, in which contributing vision problems are present. VSE and VPM skills are integral factors in the process of learning-to-read in the early school years and of reading-to-learn in later school years. Extensive discussion of these issues is presented by Stein.[108]

Summary

The acquisition of VSE and VPM functions is a developmental process that requires the child to interact with his or her environment. VPM development correlates with early academic achievement. This relation is especially compelling when analyzed by multivariate analysis. Although specific types of dyslexia, with the possible exception of dysnemkinesia, are not caused by VSE or VPM dysfunctions, they are important contributing factors in cases of dyslexia (specific RD) and as possible primary causative factors in cases of nonspecific RD. Whether or not dyslexia is present, vision therapy is a viable treatment option to improve the individual's visual information–processing ability when VSE and VPM problems either cause or contribute to the RD.

References

1. Johnson DJ, Myklebust HR. Learning Disabilities: Educational Principles and Practices. New York: Grune & Stratton, 1967.
2. Hynd GW, Cohen M. Dyslexia: Neuropsychological Theory, Research and Clinical Differentiation. New York: Grune & Stratton, 1983.
3. Solan HA, Mozlin R. Correlations of perceptual-motor maturation to readiness and reading in kindergarten and the primary grades. J Am Optom Assoc 1986;57:28–35.
4. Haynes H, White BL, Held R. Visual accommodations in human infants. Science 1965;148:528–30.
5. Brookman KE. Ocular accommodation in human infants. Ph.D. Thesis. Indiana University, 1980.
6. Schor CM, Ciufreda KJ. Vergence Eye Movements: Basic and Clinical Aspects. Boston: Butterworth, 1983;101–73.
7. Ludlam WM. The Diagnosis and Treatment of Functional Visual Disorders. In HA Solan (ed), The Treatment and Management of Children with Learning Disabilities. Springfield, IL: Thomas, 1982;119–67.
8. Pirozzolo FJ, Rayner K. The Neural Control of EM's in Acquired and Developmental Reading Disorder. In H Avakian-Whitaker, HA Whitaker (eds), Advances in Neurolinguistics and Psycholinguistics. New York: Academic, 1978.
9. Hoffman LG. Incidence of vision difficulties in children with learning disabilities. J Am Optom Assoc 1980;51:447–51.
10. Chernick B. Profile of perceptual visual anomalies in the disabled reader. J Am Optom Assoc 1978;49:1117–8.
11. Wold RM (ed). Vision, Its Impact on Learning. Seattle: Special Child Publications, 1978;96–110.
12. Sherman A. Relating vision disorders to learning disability. J Am Optom Assoc 1973;44:140–1.

13. Taylor EA. Controlled Reading: A Correlation of Diagnostic, Teaching, and Corrective Techniques. Chicago: University of Chicago Press, 1937;2.
14. Taylor EA. The spans: perception, apprehension, and recognition as related to reading and speed reading. Am J Ophthalmol 1957;44:501–7.
15. Taylor SE. Eye movements in reading: facts and fallacies. Am Educ Residency J 1965;2:4.
16. Gilbert LC. Functional Motor Efficiency of the Eyes and its Relation to Reading. Berkeley: University of California Press, 1953.
17. Tinker MA. Bases for Effective Reading. Minneapolis: University of Minnesota Press, 1965.
18. Griffin DC, Walton HN, Ives V. Saccades as related to reading disorders. J Learn Disabil 1974;7:310–6.
19. Pavlidis G. Sequencing, Eye Movements and Early Objective Diagnosis of Dyslexia. In G Pavlidis, TR Miles (eds), Dyslexia Research and Its Applications to Education. New York: Wiley, 1981;99–163.
20. Hoffman LG, Rouse MW. Referral recommendations for binocular function and/or developmental perceptual deficiencies. J Am Optom Assoc 1980;51:119–25.
21. Bennett GR, Blondin M, Ruskiewicz J. Incidence and prevalence of selected visual conditions. J Am Optom Assoc 1982;53:647–56.
22. Poynter HL, Schor C, Haynes HM, et al. Oculomotor functions in reading disability. Am J Optom Physiol Opt 1982;59:116–27.
23. Passmore JW, Maclean F. Convergence insufficiency and its management: an evaluation of 100 patients receiving a course in orthoptics. Am J Ophthalmol 1957;43:448–56.
24. Mahto RS. Eye strain from convergence insufficiency. Br Med J 1972;2:564–5.
25. Mayou S. The treatment of convergence deficiency. Br Orthoptic J 1945;3:72–82.
26. Capobianco NM. Symposium on convergence insufficiency: incidence and diagnosis. Am Orthoptic J 1953;3:13–7.
27. Rosenfeld J. Convergence insufficiency in children and adults. Am Orthoptic J 1967;17:93–7.
28. Marcus SE. A syndrome of visual constrictions in the learning disabled child. J Am Optom Assoc 1974;45:746–9.
29. Griffin JR, Grisham JD. Binocular Anomalies: Diagnosis and Vision Therapy. Boston: Butterworth-Heinemann, 1995.
30. Dunlop P. The changing role of orthoptics in dyslexia. Br Orthoptic J 1976;33:22–8.
31. Allen DDA, et al. Analysis of the Results of the Washington County District 15 Elementary School Vision Screening Program (The Abbo Study). O.D. thesis. Pacific University College of Optometry, 1975.
32. Eames TH. Comparison of eye conditions among 1000 reading failures, 500 ophthalmic patients, and 150 unselected children. Am J Ophthalmol 1948;31:713–7.
33. Park GE, Burri C. The relation of various eye conditions and reading achievement. J Educ Psychol 1943;34:290–9.
34. Robinson H, Huelsman C Jr. Visual Efficiency and Progress. In H Robinson (ed), Clinical Studies in Reading. Chicago: University of Chicago Press, 1953;49–65.

35. Benton CD. Management of Dyslexias Associated with Binocular Control Abnormalities. In AH Keeney, VT Keeney (eds), Dyslexia Diagnosis and Treatment of Reading Disorders. St. Louis: Mosby, 1968;143–54.
36. Simons HD, Grisham JD. Binocular anomalies and reading problems. J Am Optom Assoc 1987;58:578–87.
37. Simons HD, Gassler PA. Vision anomalies and reading skill: a meta-analysis of the literature. Am J Optom Physiol Opt 1988;65:893–904.
38. Evans JR, Efron M, Hodge C. Incidence of lateral phoria among SLD children. Acad Therapy 1976;11:431–3.
39. Cassin B. Strabismus and learning disabilities. Am Orthoptic J 1975;25:38–45.
40. Solan HA, Ciner EB. Visual perception and learning: issues and answers. J Am Optom Assoc, 1989;60:457–60.
41. Lyle TK. Worth and Chavasse's Squint: The Binocular Reflexes and Treatment of Strabismus. London: Bailliere, Tindall & Cox, 1950.
42. Wiesel TN, Hubel DH. Single cell responses in striate cortex of kittens deprived of vision in one eye. J Neurophysiol 1963;26:1003–17.
43. Held R. Plasticity in sensory-motor systems. Sci Am 1965;213:84–94.
44. Kratz KE, Spear PD, Smith DC. Postcritical-period reversal effects of monocular deprivation on striate cortex cells in the cat. J Neurophysiol 1976;39:501–11.
45. Singer W, Tretter F, Yinon U. Central grating of developmental plasticity in kitten visual cortex. J Physiol (Lond) 1982;324:221–37.
46. Suchoff IB. Visual-Spatial Development in the Child: An Optometric Theoretical and Clinical Approach. New York: SUNY College of Optometry, 1981.
47. Barsch RH. Achieving Perceptual-Motor Efficiency (Perceptual Motor Curriculum; Vol 1). Seattle: Special Child Publications, 1967.
48. Gesell A, Ilg F, Bulles G. Vision: Its Development in Infant and Child. New York: Paul B Hoeber, 1949;81.
49. Piaget J, Inhelder B. The Child's Conception of Space. New York: Norton Library, 1967.
50. Getman GN. How to Develop Your Child's Intelligence. Wayne, PA: Research Publications, 1962.
51. McAninch M. Body Image as Related to Perceptual-Cognitive-Motor Disabilities. In J Hellmuth (ed), Learning Disorders, Vol 2. Seattle: Special Child Publications, 1966;144.
52. Early GH. Perceptual Training in the Curriculum. Columbus, OH: Charles E Merrill, 1969;15.
53. Cron M. Overview of Normal Child Development. In MM Scheiman, MW Rouse (eds), Optometric Management of Learning-Related Vision Problems. St. Louis: Mosby, 1994;3–34.
54. Cratty BJ. Perceptual and Motor Development in Infants and Children (3rd ed). Englewood Cliffs, NJ: Prentice-Hall, 1986.
55. Piaget J. Judgment and Reasoning in the Child. New York: Harcourt, Brace, 1928;290.
56. Benton AL. Right-Left Discrimination and Finger Localization: Development and Pathology. New York: Harper & Row, 1959.
57. Gardner MF. Test of Visual Perceptual Skills (TVPS). Burlingame, CA: Psychological & Educational Publications, 1982.
58. Solan HA (ed), The Treatment and Management of Children with Learning Disabilities. Springfield, IL: Thomas, 1982.

59. Coleman HM. The West Warwich visual perception study—part 1. J Am Optom Assoc 1972;43:452–62.
60. Solan HA. The effects of visual-spatial and verbal skills on written and mental arithmetic. J Am Optom Assoc 1987;58:88–94.
61. Gesell A, Ilg FL. The Child from Five to Ten. New York: Harper & Row, 1946;427.
62. Keogh, BK. Optometric vision training programs for children with learning disabilities: review of issues and research. J Learn Disabil 1974;7:219–31.
63. Gibson JJ, Gibson EJ. Perceptual learning: differentiation or enrichment. Psychol Rev 1955;62:32–41.
64. Ginsburg GP, Hartwick A. Directional confusion as a sign of dyslexia. Percept Mot Skills 1971;32:535–43.
65. Lovell K, Gorton A. A study of some differences between backward readers of average intelligence as assessed by a non-verbal test. Br J Educ Psychol 1968;38:240–8.
66. Monk ES. Reading Reversal, Right-Left Discrimination and Lateral Preferences. Ph.D. dissertation. Columbia University, 1966.
67. Kaufman NL. Review of research on reversal errors. Percept Mot Skills 1980;51:55–79.
68. Brunswick E. Perception and the Representative Design of Psychological Experiments. Berkeley: University of California Press, 1956.
69. O'Neil WM. Basic issues in perceptual theory. Psychol Rev 1958;65:348–61.
70. Barrett TC. Review: visual discrimination and first grade reading. Reading Res Q 1965;1:51–76.
71. Smith NB. Matching ability as a factor in first grade reading. J Educ Psychol 1928;19:560–71.
72. Lee JM, et al. Measuring reading readiness. Elementary School J 1958;140:25–36.
73. Gates AI. An experimental evaluation of reading readiness tests. Elementary School J 1939;39:497–508.
74. Olson AV. Growth in word perception abilities as it relates to success in beginning reading. J Educ 1958;140:25–36.
75. Gavel SR. June reading achievements of 1st grade children. J Educ 1958;140:37–43.
76. Cruickshank WM, et al. Perception and Cerebral Palsy. Syracuse: Syracuse University Press, 1957.
77. Fildes LG. A psychological inquiry into the nature of the condition known as congenital word-blindness. Brain 1921;44:286.
78. Orton ST. Reading, Writing and Speech Problems in Children. New York: Norton, 1937.
79. Lyle JG, Goyen J. Visual recognition, developmental lag, and strephosymbolia in reading retardation. J Abnorm Psychol 1968;73:25–9.
80. Whipple CI, Kodman F Jr. A study of discrimination and perceptual learning with retarded readers. J Educ Psychol 1969;60:1–5.
81. Myklebust HR, Johnson D. Dyslexia in children. Except Child 1962;29:14–25.
82. Bakker DJ. Temporal Order in Disturbed Reading. Rotterdam: Rotterdam University Press, 1971.
83. Morrison FJ, Giordani B, Nagy J. Reading disability: an information processing analysis. Science 1977:196:77–9.

84. Mason M. Reading ability and letter search time: effects of orthographic structure defined by single-letter positional frequency. J Exp Psychol Gen 1975;104:146–66.
85. O'Neill G, Stanley G. Visual processing of straight lines in dyslexic and normal children. Br J Educ Psychol 1976;46:323–7.
86. Frostig M. Visual perception, integrative functions and academic learning. J Learn Disabil 1972;5:1–15.
87. Koppitz EM. The Bender Gestalt Test for Young Children. New York: Grune & Stratton, 1963.
88. Silver A. Diagnostic considerations in children with reading disability. Bull Orton Soc 1961;11:5–12.
89. Epstein HR. The Role of Haptic and Performatory Activity on Visual Perception in Young Children. Paper presented at the 9th Annual International Interdisciplinary UAP Conference on Piagetian Theory, Feb. 3, 1979.
90. Netley C. Prismatic adaptation and visuo-motor skills in children with learning disabilities. J Learn Disabil 1973;6:377–82.
91. Ryckman DB, Rentfrow RK. The Beery Developmental Test of Visual-Motor Integration: an investigation of reliability. J Learn Disabil 1971;4:333–4.
92. Beery KE. Visual-Motor Integration Test. Chicago: Follett, 1967. (Revised VMI available from Vision Extension, Santa Ana, CA 92705.)
93. Ames LB. Children with perceptual problems may also lag developmentally. J Learn Disabil 1969;2:205–8.
94. Satz P, Spanow S. Specific Developmental Dyslexia: A Theoretical Reformulation. In DJ Bakker, P Satz (eds), Specific Reading Disability: Advances in Theory and Method. Rotterdam: Rotterdam University Press, 1970;17–40.
95. Satz P, Rardin D, Ross J. An evaluation of a theory of specific developmental dyslexia. Child Dev 1971;42:2009–21.
96. Satz P, Von Nostrand GK. Developmental Dyslexia: An Evaluation of a Theory. In P Satz, JJ Ross (eds), The Disabled Learner: Early Detection and Intervention. Rotterdam: Rotterdam University Press, 1973.
97. Satz P, Friel J. Some predictive antecedents of specific reading disability: a preliminary 2-year follow-up. J Learn Disabil 1974;7:437–44.
98. Gibson EJ. Learning to Read. In NS Endler (ed), Contemporary Issues in Developmental Psychology. New York: Rinehart, 1968;291–303.
99. Luria AR. Higher Cortical Functions in Man. New York: Basic Books, 1966.
100. Weiner PS, Wepman JM. The relationship of early perceptual level functioning to later school achievements in block disadvantaged child. Div Res Demonst Grants SRS, Dept of HEW, Washington, D.C., 1971.
101. Velluntino FR. Dyslexia. Sci Am 1987;256:34–41.
102. Griffin JR, Birch TF, Bateman GF. Dyslexia and visual perception: is there a relation. Optom Vis Sci 1993;70:374–9.
103. Griffin JR, Walton HN. Dyslexia Determination Test (DDT) (rev ed). Los Angeles: Instructional Materials and Equipment Distributors, 1987.
104. Do N, Lo A, Griffin JR. The Performance of Dysphonetic Dyslexics on the Test of Visual Perceptual Skills. Research Project, 1992, copy in the M.B. Ketchum Memorial Library of the Southern California College of Optometry, Fullerton, CA.

105. Solan HA, Ficarra AP. A study of perceptual and verbal skills of disabled readers in grades 4, 5 and 6. J Am Optom Assoc 1990;61:628–34.
106. Solan HA, Groffman S. Developmental and Perceptual Assessment of Learning-Disabled Children: Theoretical Concepts and Diagnostic Testing. Santa Ana, CA: Optometric Extension Program Foundation, 1994;11–3.
107. Groffman S. The Relationship Between Visual Perception and Learning. In MM Scheiman, MW Rouse (eds), Optometric Management of Learning-Related Vision Problems. St. Louis: Mosby, 1994;197–208.
108. Stein JF (ed). Vision and Visual Dyslexia. Boca Raton, FL: CRC Press, 1991.

7 Eye Movement Control and Reading

Eye movement control is a complex interaction between lower levels of visual processing and higher-level cortical output. In this chapter, the eye movements involved in the process of reading are discussed; other aspects of binocular control are covered in Chapters 9 and 11.

Saccades

In reading, eye movements are necessary for the continuing acquisition and updating of visually presented information. For the most part, eye movements can be categorized into two basic systems: pursuits and saccades. Pursuits (following movements) require constant target foveation. Saccades are rapid eye movements estimated to take place about 250,000 times per day.[1] Every saccade requires an eye movement together with a fixation pause each time the object of interest comes to rest on the fovea. Information processing occurs during this time. Between fixations, when the eyes are moving, the brain does not process information.[2] The eye registers no awareness of a blurred image, even though the visual world is rapidly sweeping across the retina—a phenomenon referred to as saccadic omission. Saccadic omission is aided by two other processes: saccadic suppression (the threshold for detection of light is elevated during a saccade) and visual masking, which is generated by a highly contoured visual environment present before and after the saccade. The mechanism for saccadic suppression and visual masking appears to be within the striate cortex and superior colliculus.[3–5]

In reading, saccades are the most significant eye movement skill. Saccades are driven by rapid, high-frequency bursts of neural activity producing high-speed ocular acceleration. During these brief periods of saccadic activity, antagonist muscle action is turned off, only to be reactivated when the fovea reaches the object of interest. Even with antagonistic muscle reactivation, several types of foveal "overshooting" can occur when the fovea oversteps the target of regard. There are three distinct forms of overshooting. The first, present in normal eye movements, is known as dynamic overshoot. This high-speed overshoot lasts but a few milliseconds before the fovea returns to the target. This type of overshoot cannot be observed by the clinician without the aid of special eye movement monitors. The second type of overshoot is glissadic overshoot: the eye oversteps the target and then makes a relatively slow gliding motion back to the target, taking about 200 milliseconds. In our opinion, a trained clinician can often observe such a return, although some researchers claim it cannot be seen without the use of a recording device. The third type is static overshoot: The eye remains in a fixed position beyond the target for 150–200 milliseconds before the return. This type of overshoot is usually easy to observe and is considered pathognomonic of cerebellar dysfunction.[6]

In the normal act of reading, each forward saccade (reading from left-to-right for English and many other languages) is followed by a fixational pause that lasts 200–250 milliseconds, during which information is obtained about the word or word phrase. A normal fixation acquires 6–8 characters of text within the foveal region, which is represented by a 2-degree central area at normal viewing distances. This area of information processing is often referred to as the perceptual span of recognition. There have been many attempts to measure this perceptual span. Different methods have yielded varying results. In general, the perceptual span of skilled readers extends from 3–4 letters to the left of fixation to approximately 15 characters to the right.[7] Of that 19-character span, word identification occurs within a 9-character zone that extends 3–4 characters to the left of fixation and 5–6 characters to the right (Figure 7.1). Rayner[8] suggested that there are three perceptual spans, one each for letters, words, and total perception. The presence of these different perceptual spans for reading complicates the research picture because the size of the span influences the length of the saccade. What seems evident is that, in the reading act, each successive saccade has an overlapping perceptual span from the previous fixation.

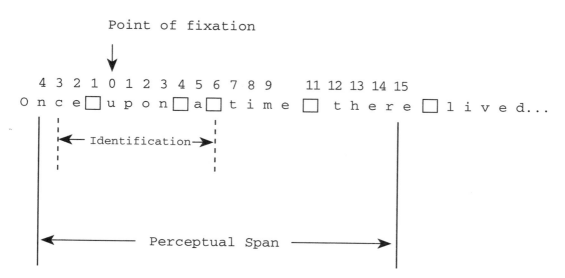

FIGURE 7.1 *Diagram illustrating perceptual span and zone of identification in reading.*

During a saccade, because of saccadic suppression, no information is derived from the printed text. Beginning readers may require more than one fixation per word, whereas older, more experienced readers require fewer saccades and fixations. Saccades during reading are not always progressive (forward). They may be regressive (backward) and are thought to be used to reread words or to verify what was previously read. Regressions generally occupy 5–20% of all saccadic activity during reading.[1] Faster readers have shorter durations of fixation, longer saccades, and fewer regressions than do slower readers.[8] When the eyes reach the end of a line of print, there is a large regressive movement to the next line, known as a return sweep, which is also classified as a saccade.

Poor Saccades and Reading Dysfunction

Given the relative precision required for saccades, the complexity of the reading process, and the physiology of eye movements, it seems logical to assume that reading behaviors can be easily disrupted if the saccadic system is dysfunctional. Many investigators have studied the relation between saccades and individuals with reading problems. The research is confusing as to cause and effect. It is uncertain how much of an adverse effect poor eye movement control has on reading. Saccadic precision, however, is particularly important in the first few years of school because the reading process is generally performed word by word, or perhaps letter by letter, rather than in word phrases.

In the normal reading process, acquisition of information requires matching of oral language with that of the written language code. Difficulty with the language aspects of reading may masquerade as an eye movement dysfunction. For example, losing place when reading may not be a sign of poor eye movement control; rather, it may be due to difficulty in matching language with the text as the coded information is processed and reprocessed.

As text difficulty increases, fixation duration increases, saccadic length decreases, and the number of regressions increases[7] (Figure 7.2). Other factors also influence the saccadic interval. Rayner[9] and O'Regan[10] demonstrated that, in the process of reading, fixation on a word is not random; rather, the preferred location for fixation is between the beginning and middle letters of the word. Furthermore, there is evidence that the length of the upcoming word influences the length of the saccadic movement.[11] Researchers have demonstrated that poor readers have eye movement patterns that mimic increases in text difficulty; there are more fixations per line, longer durations of fixation, shorter saccades, and more regressions.[12–15] Consequently, it may be the nature of the cognitive process when attempting to break the written code that is secondarily causing poor eye movement control rather than the presence of a primary eye movement problem.

Temporal Processing and Eye Movement Control

Although the eye movement physiology may be intact in all but a few individuals who have significant ocular pathology, accuracy in reading may be adversely influenced by a defective temporal-processing mechanism. As pointed out in Chapters 4 and 5, the visual system processes both spatial and temporal information. The temporal nature of vision is reflected in movement detection and plays an important role in the reading process because eye position information is constantly updated during reading. Breitmeyer and Ganz[16] and others have hypothesized that the temporal component of the visual system inhibits visible persistence during the act of reading (see Chapter 5). That is, with each new saccade, the previously fixated text must be erased from the precognitive (low-level) aspects of the visual system. If this were not the case, the text afterimage would persist and "bleed" into the image produced by the next fixation, when additional text is foveated. As with a piano, if there is no damping mechanism to eliminate the tone of the struck piano key, its sound persists into the next note played. Such a damping mechanism is hypothesized for the visual system to prevent a carryover (visible persistence) of the previously fixated image.

Individuals who display difficulty with eye movement control may have a temporal-processing deficit. Clinical testing using traditional

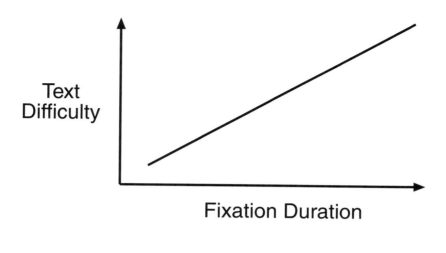

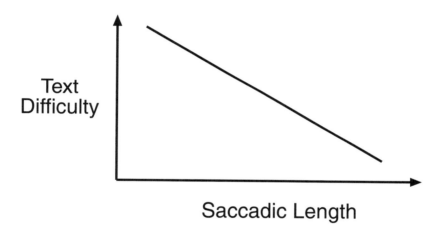

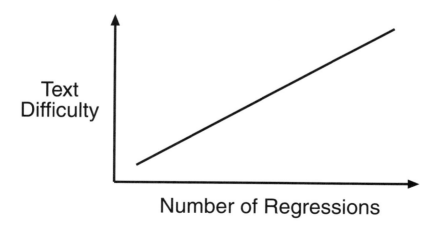

FIGURE 7.2 *Effect of text difficulty on fixation duration, saccadic length, and number of regressions during reading.*

methods, such as having the patient visually track an object or fixate from one object to another, cannot be expected to uncover a temporal deficit. Unfortunately, there is no quick and practical clinical test for this purpose. We speculate, however, that a temporal-processing deficit may be presumed through exclusionary diagnosis, consisting of a careful case history and a series of clinical rule-out testing procedures.

Patients with temporal-processing deficits may report any of the following symptoms: (1) movement of words on a printed page, (2) words or letters "running together," (3) ghostlike doubling of letters and words, (4) nauseated feeling accompanied by word movement, (5) loss of place, (6) skipping lines, (7) ill-sustained concentration, and (8) unintentional rereading of words. These symptoms are similar to the *scotopic sensitivity syndrome* proposed by Irlen.[17] Although any or all of these symptoms may suggest a temporal-processing deficit, these symptoms are most often related to either refractive, accommodative, vergence, or primary eye movement dysfunction, or combinations thereof for which vision therapy is efficacious.[18]

Eye Movement Dysfunction and Allocation of Attention

Allocation of attention, also known as on-task looking behavior or vigilance, may play a significant role in the accuracy of eye movements. Behaviors that might normally be attributed to primary eye movement–control dysfunction may represent a problem of attention allocation. Richman suggests that measuring on-task looking behavior can be an important differential diagnostic sign for the presence of physiologic or pathologic eye movement–control dysfunction.[19] Readers who have problems maintaining their place on the page or losing comprehension when reading may have problems with attention. The primary purpose in the creation of the Developmental Eye Movement test (DEM) was to differentiate individuals with eye movement–control dysfunction from those with verbal automaticity problems.[20] We believe, however, that the DEM can also be used to detect an attentional problem. Poor attentional behavior is indicated when the subject has as much difficulty calling out the numbers in the vertical columns as in the horizontal rows. The time and error scores for both vertical and horizontal presentations is likely to be poor.

Differentiating between automaticity and attentional difficulty is probably not possible using the DEM as it is now administered and scored. Richman subsequently developed a computerized test (available from Bernell Corporation[21]) to measure vigilance. This test uses a timed, successively presented series of letters located in the same position on a computer screen. The patient's task is to press a key every time he or she sees the letter X. On-task looking behavior can then be measured. Comparison of performance on the DEM with this vigilance task can eliminate the ambiguity of the DEM in differentiating automaticity from attentional problems. If attentional problems are present, the patient is likely to perform poorly on both tasks. If the patient has only automaticity difficulty, he or she will do better spotting the X targets on the vigilance test than when calling out the numbers on the DEM.

Dyslexia Related to Eye Movements

Dyslexic readers tend to have eye movements with longer fixation duration, shorter saccadic length, and greater number of regressions than normal readers.[7, 12–15] These eye movement characteristics of dyslexic readers appear similar to those of normal readers when attempting to read a relatively difficult text (see Figure 7.2). The question is whether dyslexia is the result or the cause of faulty eye movements. We believe that dyslexia is not caused by eye movement problems. We contend, however, that faulty eye movement control has an adverse effect on reading efficiency, regardless of whether the individual is dyslexic or nondyslexic.

Dyslexia may be the principal reason for longer fixations, often because additional time is needed for word recognition. A dyseidetic reader relies heavily on phonetic decoding, which is slower than eidetic decoding. A dysphonetic reader is naturally poor in word-attack skills, thus making phonetic decoding even slower. Shorter saccadic lengths may be the result of the need to syllabicate, particularly for a dyseidetic. An excessive number of regressions may be necessary for the dyslexic reader to double-check previously decoded words for correctness. For example, "The boy went to the horse and got on it for a ride." The dyslexic reader may have incorrectly identified *horse* as *house*, but later, through contextual analysis, realized the decoding error.

Are any subtypes of dyslexia associated with faulty eye movements in reading? This is a difficult question to answer, mainly because subtypes have not been clearly defined in many research reports (see Chapters 1–3 and 10 for discussions of subtyping). Morris and Rayner[7] discussed the possible relation of eye movement behavior in terms of three proposed subgroups of dyslexia: (1) general language deficit (the vast majority of dyslexics), (2) visual-spatial deficit (a much smaller group of dyslexics), and (3) selective attentional deficit. Their conclusions on the role of eye movements were not definitive because of contradictions on both sides of the issue. In general, however, the consensus was that individuals with general language deficits tend to have readings levels similar to those of younger normal readers. An argument they cited against this classification was that "there are many components of language processing that could be at the root of the difficulties experienced by such dyslexics." Their second type (visual-spatial dyslexics) demonstrated a tendency to move their eyes to the left more frequently than normal in both reading and nonreading tasks. We have seen no clinical evidence of this in dyseidetic or dysphonetic patients on electronically recorded ophthalmographic tests of saccadic skills. Of course, regressions due to poor decoding would cause the eyes to move to the left. Regressions occur in dyslexia, regardless of the subtype. The third type (selective attentional deficit dyslexia) is speculative and lacks clinical and research support (see Chapter 1, under Causes of Reading Dysfunction, on attentional problems being a general contributory cause of reading dysfunction).

Grisham and Simons[22] suggested a possible relation between dyseidesia and "oculomotor sequential deficiencies" but no relation between the latter and dysphonesia. We are concerned that dyseidesia was equated with the visual-spatial subgroup of Morris and Rayner,[7] and dysphonesia was equated with "the more prevalent auditory-linguistic subgroup." Grisham and Simons commented on a study by Brown et al.[23] that contradicted the conclusion of Pavlidis[15] by finding no primary eye movement–control problem. According to Grisham and Simons, the study by Brown et al. "was particularly well-designed and had a well-matched control group for the dyslexic subjects. Judging from the dyslexic selection criteria, though, it appears that the dyslexias were all of the *dysphonetic* [our emphasis] type." Griffin reviewed the data of Brown et al. and could not confirm that all dyslexic subjects had dysphonesia. Also, it is unlikely that any large sample of dyslexic subjects would be composed of only one type of dyslexia. Furthermore, there is insufficient evidence to equate dyseidesia with the visual-spatial subgroup or dysphonesia with the auditory-linguistic subgroup either clinically or for research purposes. Nevertheless, the insights of Grisham and Simons are of value in that differences in eye movement behavior may exist when comparing the several directly diagnosed types of dyslexia.

We are unable to differentiate dyseidesia from dysphonesia on the basis of eye movement behavior. Our clinical experience, however, has led us to believe that patients with dysphoneidesia (the more serious, mixed type) tend to have slightly more eye movement control problems than do normal readers. This may also be true when comparing dysphoneidesia to either dyseidesia or dysphonesia alone. A study by Wesson[24] found a statistically significant difference between the dysphoneidetics and dyseidetics. The sample size for dysphonesia was too small to evaluate for statistical purposes. Wesson's results are not surprising because dysphoneidetic individuals may show signs or symptoms of other associated problems, such as magnocellar defects[25] or visual-motor dysfunction.[26] We propose that a cause of the widespread effect in dysphoneidesia is that both Wernicke's area and the angular gyrus are involved; there may be a cluster of neurologic dysfunctions that "spill over" to other portions of the brain. Eye movement control centers, therefore, could also be involved. An excellent book by Ciuffreda and Tannen discusses eye movements in great detail.[27]

Summary

Adequate eye movement control is necessary for efficient reading. As text becomes more cognitively demanding (or difficult in other ways, such as from poor quality print), the reader makes more fixations with shorter saccades and has more regressions. Poor readers, from whatever cause or causes, may show similar eye movement behavior with relatively less text demands. Efficient reading may be affected adversely by a defective temporal-processing mechanism; this should be ruled out to the extent feasible. Likewise, attentional and automaticity problems affecting eye movements should be evaluated. Eye movement problems do not seem to cause dyslexia, although there may be a significant correlation with dysphoneidetic dyslexia.

References

1. Stark LW, Giveen SC, Terdiman JF. Specific Dyslexia and Eye Movements. In JF Stein (ed), Vision and Visual Dyslexia. Boca Raton, FL: CRC Press, 1991;203–32.
2. Leigh RJ, Zee DS. The Neurology of Eye Movements (2nd ed). Philadelphia: FA Davis, 1991;86.
3. Judge SJ, Wurtz RH, Richmond BJ. Vision during saccadic eye movements: visual interactions in the striate cortex. J Neurophysiol 1980;43:1133–55.
4. Richmond BJ, Wurtz RH. Vision during saccadic eye movements: a corollary discharge to monkey superior colliculus. J Neurophysiol 1980;43:1156–67.
5. Wurtz RH, Albano JE. Visual-motor function of the primate superior colliculus. Annu Rev Neurosci 1980;3:189–226.
6. Bahill AT, Stark L. Trajectories of saccadic eye movements. Sci Am 1979;240:108–17.
7. Morris RK, Rayner K. Eye Movements in Skilled Reading: Implications for Developmental Dyslexia. In JF Stein (ed), Vision and Visual Dyslexia. Boca Raton, FL: CRC Press, 1991;233–42.
8. Rayner K. Eye movements in reading and information processing. Psychol Bull 1978;85:618–60.
9. Rayner K. Eye guidance in reading: fixation location within words. Perception 1979;8:21–30.
10. O'Regan JK. The Convenient Viewing Position Hypothesis. In DF Fisher, RA Monty, JW Senders (eds), Eye Movements: Cognition and Visual Perception. Hillsdale, NJ: Erlbaum, 1981.
11. Morris RK, Rayner K, Pollatsek A. Eye movement guidance in reading: the role of parafoveal letter and space information. Hum Percept Perform 1990;16:268–81.
12. Rubino CA, Minden HA. An analysis of eye movements in children with a reading disability. Cortex 1973;9:217–20.
13. Pirozzolo FJ. The Neuropsychology of Developmental Reading Disorders. New York: Praeger, 1979.

14. Elterman RD, Abel LA, Daroff RB, et al. Eye movement patterns in dyslexic children. J Learn Disabil 1980;13:312–7.
15. Pavlidis GTH. The "Dyslexia Syndrome" and its Objective Diagnosis by Erratic Eye Movements. In K Rayner (ed), Eye Movements in Reading: Perceptual and Language Processes. New York: Academic, 1983;441–67.
16. Breitmeyer BG, Ganz L. Implications of sustained and transient channels for theories of visual pattern masking, saccadic suppression, and information processing. Psychol Rev 1976;83:1–36.
17. Irlen H. Successful treatment of learning disabilities. Presentation at the 91st annual meeting of the American Psychological Association, 1983.
18. Scheiman M, Blaskey P, Ciner EB, et al. Vision characteristics of individuals identified as Irlen filter candidates. J Am Optom Assoc 1990;61:600–5.
19. Richman JE. Use of sustained attention task to determine children at risk for learning problems. J Am Optom Assoc 1986;57:20–6.
20. Garzia RP, Richman JE, Nicholson SB. A new visual-verbal saccade test: the developmental eye movement test (DEM). J Am Optom Assoc 1990;61:124–35.
21. Bernell Corporation. 750 Lincolnway East, P.O. Box 4637, South Bend, IN 46634.
22. Grisham D, Simons H. Perspectives on Reading Disabilities. In AA Rosenbloom, MW Morgan (eds), Principles and Practice of Pediatric Optometry. Philadelphia: Lippincott, 1990;518–59.
23. Brown B, Haegerstrom-Portnoy G, Yingling CD, et al. Tracking eye movements are normal in dyslexic children. Am J Optom Physiol Opt 1983;60:376–83.
24. Wesson MD. Eye Movements in Dyslexia. Study at UAB School of Optometry, Birmingham, AL, 1995.
25. Ridder WH III, Borsting E. Which dyslexic subtypes demonstrate a magnocellular pathway defect? Presented at the annual meeting of the American Academy of Optometry, San Diego, Dec. 13, 1994.
26. Wesson MD. The relation between visual-perceptual skills and dyslexia. Part I. Visual-motor skills. Presented at the annual meeting of the American Academy of Optometry, San Diego, Dec. 13, 1994.
27. Ciuffreda KJ, Tannen B. Eye Movement Basics for the Clinician. St. Louis: Mosby, 1995.

8   Role of Auditory Perception

Auditory Perception Definition

Auditory perception is the identification, interpretation, and organization of sensory data received through the ear.[1] Although auditory perception may be defined in a variety of ways, it always implies higher-order (cognitive) auditory processing. This definition does not, however, exclude processing at lower (precognitive) levels of the auditory system.[2] Auditory perception and the term *central auditory processing* (CAP) are often used interchangeably, although CAP appears to be a more explicit term because, by definition, CAP includes both normal intelligence and hearing sensitivity.[3] Audiologists tend to diagnose problems of auditory processing as *central auditory processing disor-*

ders (CAPDs), whereas speech pathologists, optometrists, and others refer to *auditory-perceptual deficits* (APDs). The implication of both terms is that normal intelligence and hearing sensitivity are present. In this chapter, we use the term *auditory perception* rather than *auditory processing* because *perception* suggests comprehension and *processing* is more of a neurophysiologic term, signifying transmission of the neural stimuli from one point to another within the brain.[4] CAPD and APD are included under the umbrella of learning disabilities and encompass impairments of attention, sequential memory, discrimination, sound blending, and closure skills.[5–7] It is estimated that the prevalence of APD is 3–5% of the school-age population.[8]

Auditory-Perceptual Framework

A general framework for auditory perception is necessary before embarking on investigation of more specific areas of auditory perception. Such a framework is suggested by Silver,[9] who divides perception into four broad categories: (1) input, (2) integration, (3) memory, and (4) output.

Auditory Input

Auditory input refers to auditory acuity (analogous to visual acuity), which is the ability to hear sounds distinctly with no physical or neurologic impairment. Distorted auditory information arises from conditions such as chronic or acute ear infection (otitis media), ruptured eardrum (tympanic membrane), and congenital or acquired malformation of the physical ear. The presence of one or more of these conditions creates a degraded initial signal that impairs the auditory-perceptual process. Auditory-perceptual capabilities most affected by distortions at this level include *auditory discrimination* (ability to distinguish similarities and differences between sounds), *auditory localization* (directional location of the sound), and *auditory figure-ground perception* (the ability to separate the competing background noise from that of the pertinent auditory signal). Silver[9] suggested another APD: *auditory lag*. This presumably occurs at the precognitive level and indicates that the individual cannot process sound input as fast as individuals with normal auditory perceptual capability. Auditory lag may be similar to deficits of visual temporal processing (see Chapter 5, Low-Level Temporal Processing Deficits and Transient System Modification).

Auditory Integration

Auditory integration (the ability to integrate other sensory information, such as visual, with auditory signal) requires *sequencing, abstraction,* and *organization*.[9] Initial auditory input is processed in a serial or *sequential* fashion, much like a typist striking one key after another. The ability to reproduce what is heard or written requires good sequencing skills. An example is a spelling test in which auditory input must be matched with either written or oral output in the serial act of spelling (encoding). The second component of integration is *abstraction*, which is necessary to obtain meaning from the sequence of auditory information. Limited skills in abstraction do not allow generalizing from specific information. For example, a child who has seen a movie may be able to discuss the specifics of the movie but cannot relate the events to other movies that use a similar story line. *Organization* is the third part of auditory integration. Organizational skills permit the child to relate previously learned information to current information that has been recorded, sequenced, and understood.[9] Organization is evident in activities such as verbalizing a story line in the correct sequence.

Auditory Memory

Auditory memory relates to short- and long-term storage of auditory information. Short-term memory is used for immediate events, such as a phone number when making a call. Long-term memory retains information for longer periods. It is generally thought that short-term memory acts as a filter for long-term memory, allowing for the discarding of superfluous information before long-term storage occurs.[10]

Output

Output is the final measure of auditory-perceptual skills. It is the accuracy of information output, either spoken or written, that represents the veracity of auditory-perceptual matching (i.e., information *in* approximates information *out*). If the output disability involves speaking, it may be considered a language disability. If the output disability involves writing, a motor disability (e.g., cerebral palsy) may be a possibility.

Chronic Otitis Media and Auditory-Perceptual Deficits

Closely associated with APD is *chronic otitis media*, which refers to inflammation of the entire tubotympanic cavity, from the pharyngeal end of the eustachian tube to the air cells at the mastoid tip.[11] The basic problem with all forms of chronic otitis media is the dysfunctional eustachian tube. The eustachian tube normally opens several times a minute. It functions to ventilate the middle ear and to drain mucus along with other debris into the pharynx. Tube failure can initiate middle ear inflammation and contribute to the persistence of that inflammation.[11]

Chronic otitis media has its greatest impact on auditory perception between birth and 3 years of age. It has been associated with delays in the acquisition of language, reduced intellectual development, and educational difficulties.[12–17] Zinkus et al.[18] found significant differences between children with chronic and severe otitis media and those with relatively infrequent and mild episodes of the same condition. Significant delays were observed in the severe group for acquisition of a 4- to 10-word vocabulary and the ability to formulate and use sentences of three or more words. They also found a general intellectual deficit among children with severe otitis media compared to subjects with the milder form. The deficits were noted in measured abilities within specific subtests on the *verbal* scale of the Wechsler Intelligence Scale for Children–Revised (WISC-R),[19] including mental arithmetic, auditory sequential memory, and auditory association. Other, more stable tests of intellectual ability were not affected. Some performance abilities were selectively affected, as represented by the *performance* subtests of the WISC-R. One ability adversely affected was the visual sequencing skill assessed with the Picture Arrangement subtest. This subtest requires the examinee to construct a story in sequence using pictures. Visual-motor coordination abilities reflected within the performance scale of the WISC-R were also affected.[18] However, motor-free visual-processing skills, such as visual attention to detail, visual-spatial orientation, and visual reproduction of form, were performed adequately by children in both groups. Reading levels in the two groups were also assessed by comparing achievement levels in word recognition, spelling, and arithmetic. Significant deficiencies in word decoding and spelling skills were found in children who had severe and chronic otitis media, but no difference was noted in arithmetic computation skills between the two groups.

Updike and Thornburg[20] also investigated reading skills and auditory processing ability in children with chronic otitis media in early childhood. They evaluated two groups of 6- and 7-year-old children matched by age, gender, socioeconomic status, and receptive vocabulary. The children were screened for normal hearing function at the time of the evaluation. One group had carefully documented histories of early chronic otitis media and the other had no documented history of otitis media. The positive-history group had otitis media occuring before the age of 2 years, as verified by the medical records of their attending physicians. In addition, they had experienced at least three episodes of middle ear problems during any single year between birth and 3 years of age. There was no history of otitis media during the 12 months before collection of the data. Using the Goldman-Fristoe-Woodcock Sound Symbols Test Battery,[21] a well-standardized battery for auditory-perceptual function, Updike and Thornburg[20] were able to determine that there was a significant difference in sound analysis, sound blending, and sound mimicry between the two groups of children. The results of classroom reading inventory testing confirmed significant differences between the groups for word decoding, instructional level, and comprehension. These results strongly suggest that chronic middle ear problems before the age of 3 may have secondary effects evident later in life. Updike and Thornburg's research implies a strong relation between auditory-perceptual skills (especially those of sound mimicry, sound analysis, and sound blending), word recognition, and reading comprehension. These results are also supported by earlier research.[22, 23]

Updike and Thornburg[20] also suggested that recurrent middle ear disease in younger children should be regarded as both a health and educational problem. Early identification, aggressive medical treatment, and active language stimulation are all necessary for the young child to develop to academic potential and thus prevent learning handicaps, including reading dysfunction (RD), due to chronic otitis media.

Medical and Surgical Treatment

Otitis media is the most prevalent illness affecting the pediatric population. It is estimated that each year in the United States there are 30 million visits to pediatricians for treatment of this type of infection.[24] The peak incidence of this disease occurs between 6 and 36 months of age, and a smaller peak occurs in the 4- to 7-year-old age group. Most initial episodes of otitis media occur at approximately 6 months of age. This is about the time when infections occur due to naturally declining infant immunities. The secondary peak at 4–7 years of age coincides with the hypertrophy of adenoid tissue in the nasopharynx adjacent to the eustachian tube orifice.

There are many risk factors involved in the development of otitis media in childhood. These include a prevalence of respiratory infections in certain localities, lower economic status, cigarette smoking in the home, and other debilitating diseases that interfere with the immune system. Chronic otitis media has a devastating impact on auditory-perceptual skills. When otitis media is present, the eustachian tube is blocked, causing a reduction of air behind the eardrum. This blockage leads to a change in the curvature of the tympanic membrane surface. Stretching the tympanic membrane in this manner causes a change in the frequency responses of the membrane as sound waves impinge on its surface. This change results in reduced responses to the middle speech sound frequencies and a consequent loss of sound information, especially that related to sound blending and other auditory-perceptual skills previously mentioned.

There are three basic stages of otitis media, according to Bluestone's classification.[25] Stage 1 is *acute* otitis media, lasting up to 3 weeks. It is characterized by rapid onset and a bulging tympanic membrane that is inflamed. Stage 2 occurs if the otitis media does not resolve within the first 3 weeks and is referred to as *subacute* otitis media and is between the fourth and eighth week of the disease. The tympanic membrane remains purulent and continues to bulge slightly and even starts to retract if the pressures between the eustachian tube and the outside air equalize. Disease persisting after 8 weeks is stage 3, *chronic* otitis media. At this point, the tympanic membrane is most frequently in a retracted position and the effusion becomes thick and mucoid.

When otitis media is diagnosed, the common mode of treatment consists of aggressive antibiotic therapy.[24] Cefaclor (Ceclor) and amoxicillin clavulanate (Augmentin) have been the antibiotics of choice for the newborn population. Cefixime (Suprax) has also been used to treat otitis media. Topical antibiotics are also used for the purulent form of otitis media. Aggressive therapy must be instituted, but most otitis specialists feel that steroid therapy is not a viable alternative, especially for long-term use.

When otitis media cannot be resolved, surgery is generally recommended under the following circumstances: 5–6 episodes of otitis media in 1 year, persistence of suppurative infection despite antibiotic therapy, or persistence of an effusion for several months with effusion becoming mucoid. The most straightforward surgical procedure is myringotomy, which consists of making a small slit in the tympanic membrane to allow drainage or active removal of suppurative or mucoid material. Unfortunately, when the tympanic membrane heals, effusion often returns in a few days. Mandel et al.,[26] using a cohort of 111 children, compared the surgical procedure of myringotomy with the use of tympanostomy tubes for ventilation. Ventilation tubes are usually made of Teflon, have a small diameter, and can be fitted into the surgical incision (myringotomy) so that the opening within the tympanic membrane stays patent as long as the ventilation tube is in place. This allows for both drainage and equalization of the atmospheric pressure. Usually the tube is extruded months or years later as a result of normal growth. When this occurs, middle ear infections may return. Some patients require a series of insertions so that the ventilation tubes support normal growth and development of the middle ear. This study demonstrated that ventilation tube insertion, together with the myringotomy and drainage of the effusion, was the best surgical procedure for chronic otitis media. Cotton[27] suggested that surgery should not be performed until at least 3 months after aggressive medical therapy. Of course, surgery is not without its risks and there may be complications with ventilation tube implants. Secondary infection occurs relatively frequently, often associated with a concomitant upper respiratory tract infection or after the entrance of water into the middle ear.[24]

Adenoidectomy has also been investigated as a surgical management procedure for chronic otitis media. This procedure has its supporters, but it is not clear whether adenoidectomy results in any consistent improvement in those suffering from recurrent otitis.[28, 29] New studies, however, advocate adenoidectomy together with tympanostomy in patients with recurrent otitis media.[30, 31] This combined procedure appears effective in reducing the rate of relapse, but this is highly dependent on the type of population evaluated.

In summary, medical management of chronic otitis media is good for a relatively short period of time. When otitis becomes acute in the presence of effusion, surgical management becomes a necessity. The longer the infection is permitted to continue, the greater the risk of loss of auditory-perceptual skills.

Auditory-Perceptual Deficits and Attention-Deficit Disorder

APD and attention-deficit disorder (ADD) have much in common. Note that there may be a hyperactivity component to the ADD, thus called attention-deficit hyperactivity disorder (ADHD). Inattention, poor listening skills, and distractibility are some of the typical indications of ADD and ADHD.[32] We use the all-inclusive abbreviation of ADD/ADHD in this section because differentiation between ADD and ADHD is not always definitive. It appears that signs and symptoms of ADD/ADHD are similar to those of children with APD, but the two conditions can most likely be differentiated by careful attention to detail in the case history and clinical testing. Although the optometrist may not routinely diagnose or directly treat ADD/ADHD, screening for APD may be performed in conjunction with testing for visual-perceptual deficits. This may help to determine whether or not there is APD.

Children with ADD/ADHD have difficulty staying on task unless constantly reinforced by novel situations. Closely linked with the task is the need for constant gratification or rewards. Even with rewards, habituation occurs relatively quickly (i.e., the rewards lose their effectiveness), requiring that the child with ADD/ADHD have even closer supervision by parents and teachers. The child with ADD/ADHD also manifests inappropriate behaviors at home with families and peers. It is important to understand that ADD/ADHD is a factor in learning disability.[9] It is generally believed that 25–40% of ADD/ADHD children have specific learning disabilities that adversely affect academic achievement.[32] Other significant features of the ADD/ADHD child may include ill health, poor socialization skills, excessive aggressiveness, and antisocial behavior.

Children with APD display many behaviors similar to children with ADD/ADHD but manifest certain differences. Most of these differences concern the use of language. The child with APD has difficulty listening in the presence of background noise, poor auditory memory, difficulty with phonics and speech sound discrimination, and poor receptive and expressive language skills. Most children with APD have actually been diagnosed with some form of learning disability related

TABLE 8.1   Differentiation Between Attention-Deficit Disorder (ADD) or ADD with Hyperactivity (ADHD) and Auditory-Perceptual Deficit (APD)

ADD and ADHD characteristics
    Difficulty staying on task
    Rewards constantly required
    Inappropriate behavior
    Need for close supervision
APD characteristics
    Poor auditory discrimination, particularly with background noise
    Poor auditory memory
    Poor listening and speaking skills
    Difficulty learning phonetic coding of words. Note that APD could simulate dysphonesia or possibly cause or at least contribute to dysphonesia. APD could be one of the environmental factors in dysphonetic dyslexia because it is probably multifactorial, as opposed to dyseidesia, which is probably a single-gene autosomal dominant trait.

to language, which is the direct result of not being able to process information accurately through the auditory channel (Table 8.1).

Keller[32] suggested that children who need referral for further evaluation for APD are those with a history of chronic otitis media, some speech articulation difficulties, and poor performance on a test of auditory discrimination (see Chapter 9) with or without the presence of background noise. When these problems are associated with RD, the optometrist should consider referral for further auditory assessment.

Summary

APD must be considered when evaluating children who have RD. Auditory-perceptual skills are the basis for spoken language and are vitally important for the establishment of phoneme-grapheme relationships in the reading process. Inadequate auditory-perceptual skills adversely affect a child who is learning to read. Consultation and remediation through professionals such as teachers, audiologists, speech and language pathologists, and occupational therapists skilled in working with APD should be considered as part of any therapeutic approach. Psychologists, psychiatrists, and pediatricians should also be consulted when ADD/ADHD is suspected. Otolaryngologists should be consulted when there is a history of otitis media.

References

1. Zinkus PW, Gottlieb MI. Patterns of perceptual and academic deficits related to chronic otitis media. Pediatrics 1980;66:246–53.

2. Katz J, Stecker NA, Henderson, D. Introduction to Central Auditory Processing. In Central Auditory Processing: A Transdisciplinary View. St. Louis: Mosby, 1992;3–8.
3. Keith RW. SCAN: A Screening Test for Auditory Processing Disorders. Cleveland, OH: The Psychological Corporation, 1986.
4. Young M. Central auditory processing through the looking glass: a critical look at diagnosis and management. J Childhood Commun Disord 1985;9:31–42.
5. Barr DF. Auditory Perceptual Disorders. Springfield, IL: Thomas, 1972;3–6.
6. Chalfant JC, Scheffelin MA. Central Processing Dysfunctions in Children: A Review of Research. Monograph 9. Bethesda, MD: National Institute of Neurological Disease and Stroke, 1969;9–19.
7. Zigmond NK. Auditory Processes in Children with Learning Disabilities. In L Tarnopol (ed), Learning Disabilities: Introduction to Educational and Medical Management. Springfield, IL: Thomas, 1969;196–212.
8. Holston JT. Assessment and management of auditory processing problems in children. Outline published by University of South Alabama, Speech and Hearing Center, 2000 University Commons, Mobile, AL 36688, circa 1994.
9. Silver LB. The Misunderstood Child: A Guide for Parents of Children with Learning Disabilities (2nd ed). Blue Ridge Summit, PA: Tab, 1992.
10. Vellutino FR. Dyslexia. Sci Am 1987;256:34–41.
11. Jahn AF. Chronic otitis media: diagnosis and treatment. Med Clin North Am 1991;75:1277–91.
12. Holm VA, Kunze LH. Effects of chronic otitis media on language and speech development. Pediatrics 1969;43:833–9.
13. Downs MP. Hearing loss: definition, epidemiology and prevention. Public Health Rev 1975;4:225–380.
14. Howie VM. The otitis-prone condition. Am J Dis Child 1975;129:676–8.
15. Paradise JP. Management of middle ear effusions in infants with cleft palate. Ann Otol Rhinol Laryngol Suppl 1976;85:285–8.
16. Ling D. Rehabilitation of Cases of Deafness Secondary to Otitis Media. In A Glorig, KS Gerwin (eds), Otitis Media. Springfield IL: Thomas, 1972;249–53.
17. Kaplan GJ, Fleshman J, Bender T. Long term effects of otitis media: a ten-year cohort study of Alaskan Eskimo children. Pediatrics 1973;52:577–85.
18. Zinkus PW, Gottlieb MI, Schapiro M. Developmental and psychoeducational sequelae of chronic otitis media. Am J Dis Child 1978;132:1100–4.
19. Wechsler DL. Manual for the Wechsler Intelligence Scale for Children–Revised. New York: Psychological Corporation, 1974.
20. Updike C, Thornburg JD. Reading skills and auditory processing ability in children with chronic otitis media in early childhood. Ann Otol Rhinol Laryngol 1992;101:530–7.
21. Goldman R, Fristoe M, Woodcock R. Goldman-Fristoe-Woodcock Sound Symbols Test Battery. Circle Pines, MN: American Guidance Service, 1974.
22. Birch JG, Belmont L. Auditory-visual integration in normal and retarded readers. Am J Orthopsychiatry 1964;34:852–61.
23. Kass C. Psycholinguistic abilities of children with reading problems. Except Child 1966;32:533–9.

24. Facione N. Otitis media: an overview of acute and chronic disease. Nurse Pract 1990;15:11–22.
25. Bluestone CD. Otitis media in children. N Engl J Med 1982;306:1399–404.
26. Mandel EM, Rockette HE, Bluestone CD, et al. Efficacy of myringotomy with and without tympanostomy tubes for chronic otitis media with effusion. Pediatr Infect Dis J 1992;11:270–7.
27. Cotton RT. The surgical management of chronic otitis media with effusion. Pediatr Ann 1991;20:630–7.
28. Roydhouse N. Adenoidectomy for otitis media with mucoid effusion. Ann Otol Rhinol Laryngol Suppl 1980;89:312–5.
29. Fiellau-Nokolajsen MA, Kolajsen M, Falbe-Hansen J, et al. Adenoidectomy for middle ear disorders: a randomized controlled trial. Clin Otolaryngol 1980;5:323–7.
30. Gates GA, Avery CA, Prihoda DJ, et al. Effectiveness of adenoidectomy and typanostomy tubes in the treatment of chronic otitis media with effusion. N Engl J Med 1987;317:1444–51.
31. Maw AR. Chronic Otitis Media with Effusion and Adenotonsillectomy: A Prospective Randomized Controlled Study. In DJ Lim (ed), Recent Advances in Otitis Media: Proceedings of the Third International Symposium, May 17–20, 1983. Philadelphia: Decker, 1984:299–303.
32. Keller WD. Auditory Processing Disorder or Attention-Deficit Disorder? In J Katz, NA Stecker, D Henderson (eds). Central Auditory Processing: A Transdisciplinary View. St. Louis: Mosby, 1992:107–14.

III. Clinical Testing

9 Evaluation of Binocular and Perceptual Skills for Vision-Related Reading Dysfunction

There are many causes of reading dysfunction (RD), some of which are the result of vision problems.[1-5] For simplicity, these vision problems can be classified as poor visual skills efficiency (VSE) and visual-perceptual-motor (VPM) skills. In an extensive review of the research on this subject, it was reported that most of these vision problems can be partially or totally eliminated with direct optometric intervention.[1] Rationales, sample testing procedures, and diagnostic evaluations are presented in this chapter (therapy is covered in Chapter 11). Topics are organized by system, proceeding from eye movements to accommodative and vergence skills to evaluation of VPM skills. As a general rule, proper development of VPM skills is most important *before* the second grade (learning to read) and the binocular skills, including oculomotor, accommodative, and vergence efficiency, are important *after* the second grade (reading to learn). In clinical practice, however, testing and evaluation of VSE skills will almost always precede that of VPM skills. Further details and information can be found in the cited references pertaining to each test discussed.

Oculomotor Skills

The evaluation of VSE should include testing of eye movements (the role of eye movements in the reading process is discussed in detail in Chapter 7). Testing of oculomotor skills pertinent to reading should include saccadic eye movements, pursuit eye movements, and fixation ability (Table 9.1).

Saccadic Eye Movements

Gross and fine saccadic eye movements should be evaluated. Although many methods can be used to assess these visual skills, we discuss the gross pencil saccade test[6] and the Developmental Eye Movement test (DEM)[7] because they are commonly used and readily available, with standardized testing and scoring.

The gross pencil saccade test requires two pencils, with a target of approximately 20/80 Snellen acuity demand at 40 cm printed on each pencil. The pencils are separated horizontally by approximately 25 cm, and the patient is instructed to fixate each target on the command of the clinician. These commands should continue for approximately 1 minute for the right eye only (left eye occluded), 1 minute for the left eye only (right eye occluded), and 1 minute for binocular testing. The patient is watched for any persistent head movements (used to assist the eye movements) and obvious undershooting or overshooting, which indicate abnormal performance. Professional judgment must always be used when evaluating such visual skills as saccadic eye movements.

The DEM provides an indirect assessment of fine saccadic eye movements, which are necessary for the act of reading. The use of

TABLE 9.1   Visual Skills Related to Reading with Testing Methods and Results Criteria

Visual Skill	Testing Method	Abnormal Finding
Gross saccades	Direct observation	Head movements, gross over- or undershooting[a]
Fine saccades	DEM	<36th percentile
Pursuits	Direct observation	>1 fixation loss
Fixations	Direct observation	Steadiness <5 secs[b]
Relative accommodation	PRA	Worse than −1.75 D
Relative accommodation	NRA	Worse than +1.75 D
Facility of accommodation	Binocular lens rock	<6 cpm with ±2.00 D[c]
Accuracy of accommodation	MEM	>+0.75 D lag or any lead[d]
Sufficiency of accommodation	Push-up amplitude	>2.00 D worse than expected for age[e]
Relative vergence	NRC at 40 cm	Blur <11$^\Delta$, break <19$^\Delta$, recovery <11$^\Delta$
Relative vergence	PRC at 40 cm	Blur <16$^\Delta$, break <20$^\Delta$, recovery <11$^\Delta$
Facility of vergence	8BI/8BO test at 40 cm	<5 cpm[f]
Accuracy of vergence	Fixation disparity	>1 min of arc (y intercept)[g]

DEM = developmental eye movement test; PRA = positive relative accommodation; NRA = negative relative accommodation; MEM = monocular estimate method retinoscopy; NRC = negative relative convergence; PRC = positive relative convergence; 8BI/8BO = 8$^\Delta$ base-in and 8$^\Delta$ base-out; cpm = cycles per minute.
[a]Or if increased latency (abnormally slow).
[b]Or if hand support needed to maintain fixation.
[c]Testing done with vectographic suppression checks.
[d]Lag of +1.00 D or more is failing and lead of −0.25 D or more is failing.
[e]Determine by Hofstetter formula: minimum amplitude = 15 − (0.25 × patient's age).
[f]Testing done with vectographic suppression monitors.
[g]Or if abnormal shape or slope of the forced vergence fixation disparity curve or if there is an abnormally high associated phoria (e.g., x intercept >5$^\Delta$).

decoding skills is minimized by using numbers, rather than words, for test stimuli. The DEM consists of (1) a number knowledge pretest, (2) two sets of vertical column arrays of numbers to assess verbal number-naming automaticity, and (3) a scattered array of numbers in horizontal rows to simulate eye movements used in reading. The pretest allows the clinician to determine whether a young child has sufficient number knowledge to perform reliably on testing. Subtests A and B present similar arrays of numbers in two vertical columns. The patient is instructed to call out each number in the first column from top to bottom and then continue to the second column. The patient is told to call out the numbers as quickly and accurately as possible. This portion of the testing is timed for speed and evaluated for any errors (omissions, additions, transpositions, and substitutions). Administration of subtest C (horizontal rows of numbers) is similar to that of subtests A and B except that the patient is to call out the numbers from left to right, row by row.

Performance time is recorded for both vertical tests (A and B) and then for the horizontal test (C). Results are evaluated individually for accuracy and speed. The horizontal time must be adjusted for any addition or omission errors. A ratio is formed by dividing the horizontal time by the sum of the vertical times. The DEM instruction manual gives expected performance times for age and grade levels. Percentile ranking can be used to determine whether the scores are abnormal (i.e., lower than the 36th percentile). Normative data for errors are also provided to assess performance.

Pursuit Eye Movements

Smooth and accurate pursuit eye movements are relatively unimportant in the act of reading, unless the individual or the printed material is moving. Trying to read a highway sign while driving an automobile, for example, would be difficult if the individual has poor pursuits. Screening of pursuit ability can be performed at 40 cm with a target equivalent to a 20/80 Snellen letter. The target should be moved at a rate of approximately 20 degrees per second in the horizontal, vertical, and diagonal directions. This testing is performed for 10 seconds. The patient is instructed to follow the target as accurately as possible. If two or more fixation losses occur during the procedure, pursuit ability is considered below normal.[6]

Fixations

Screening for fixation ability can be done at 40 cm quickly and simply by having the patient look at a target equivalent to a 20/80 Snellen letter for 10 seconds. Steadiness of fixation is judged monocularly and binocularly. Fixation ability is considered abnormal if steady fixation cannot be maintained for at least 5 seconds.[6]

Accommodative Skills

The accommodative system plays a significant role in the reading process. When accommodation is efficient, it allows for clear, comfortable vision during prolonged near work, such as reading. Hoffman and Rouse[8] related asthenopic symptoms to several accommodative dysfunctions. Of these, we discuss accommodative infacility, reduced relative accommodation, accommodative inaccuracy, and accommodative insufficiency.

Accommodative Facility

Accommodative facility is defined as the rate at which accommodation can be stimulated and inhibited repeatedly during a specific period of time.[8] Hennessey et al.[9] demonstrated that subjects with asthenopic symptoms had significantly worse than normal performance on monocular and binocular accommodative facility testing.

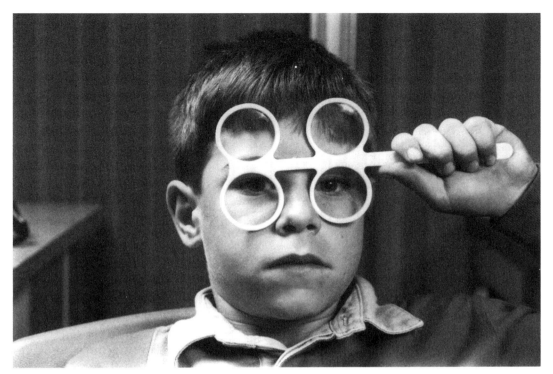

FIGURE 9.1 *Lens flipper used in testing of accommodative facility.*

Testing of nonpresbyopic patients can be performed with an appropriate lens flipper (Figure 9.1). For binocular testing, a target to monitor suppression should be used, for example, viewing the SO/V9 Acuity Suppression Slide (Bernell Corporation, South Bend, IN) (Figure 9.2) at 40 cm while wearing crossed-polarizing filters. Testing is performed with the patient's ametropia fully corrected with lenses (if the patient is not emmetropic) while +2.00 D and –2.00 D lenses are introduced alternately. Once the clinician has ascertained that the patient can clear both lens powers, the patient is told to fixate the letters pointed to by the clinician. The patient is to say the letter aloud when it is seen clearly. Testing continues for 1 minute; the number of fixations called out correctly divided by two is the accommodative facility rate in cycles per minute (cpm). The patient is alerted to monitor suppression (i.e., disappearance of any letters). The normative study by Zellers et al.[10] indicated an average of 8 cpm for binocular accommodative facility. We feel that facility less than 6 cpm is a criterion for inadequate performance (see Table 9.1).

Accommodative Accuracy

Dynamic retinoscopy is used to judge the patient's accommodative response to a nearpoint stimulus. Many techniques are used to per-

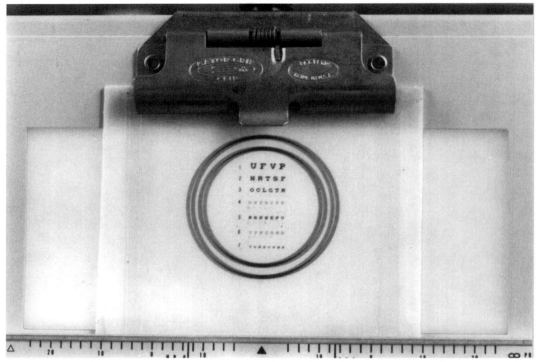

FIGURE 9.2 *Vectographic target using crossed-polarizing filters to monitor suppression when testing accommodative facility.*

form dynamic retinoscopy. Monocular estimate method (MEM) retinoscopy, first described by Haynes,[11] controls the physical and optical variables of measurement error that result from performing off-axis retinoscopy. Haynes reported better control of the sources of error than that of other dynamic retinoscopy methods, and this was confirmed by Rouse et al.,[12] who found that MEM response measurements correlated well with haploscopic measurements for accommodative stimulus levels up to 3.00 D. We recommend using MEM retinoscopy to determine the accommodative posture while performing a nearpoint task that simulates reading.

To perform MEM retinoscopy, the patient must read words held at his habitual working distance. The words are of the print size and difficulty appropriate for the patient's reading level and are closely clustered around a 1.5-cm hole in the center of the card that is held or attached to the retinoscope. This test is ideally performed with the illumination level and patient's posture simulating normal reading conditions. Furthermore, the patient should wear his or her refractive correction if it is habitually worn for reading. The MEM test may also be performed to assess the accommodative response with a tentative lens prescription to be used while reading.

The technique, performed at the patient's measured reading distance, requires retinoscopic evaluation of the horizontal meridian of each eye while the patient reads the words aloud from the card. Lenses are interposed quickly (≤1 second) to find the neutralizing lens for each eye. If MEM lag (underaccommodating) findings are greater than +0.75 D, the accommodative accuracy is abnormal.[13] Also, any lead (overaccommodating) of −0.25 D or more indicates abnormal accommodative accuracy.[6]

Relative Accommodation

The term *relative accommodation* describes the testing condition when accommodation is varied while convergence is stable. Positive relative accommodation (PRA) is the apparent increase of accommodation by adding minus lenses at the nearpoint without a change in vergence demand. Conversely, testing of negative relative accommodation (NRA) is performed with plus lenses, whereby accommodation is apparently decreased while the demand on vergence is kept constant.

Testing of PRA is performed at 40 cm with the best optical correction of ametropia and a near-threshold visual acuity target. Lenses are added in steps of −0.25 D, at approximately 2-second intervals, while the patient is instructed to keep the letters clear. The patient is instructed to report when the letters first appear blurred and remain so as testing proceeds. For nonpresbyopic patients, this should be a net of at least −1.75 D.[6] Testing is identical for NRA, but plus lenses are added until first blur is reported. This endpoint should be a net of at least +1.75 D.[6] Abnormal performance is present if the NRA or PRA is less than the expected endpoints.

Accommodative Sufficiency

The amplitude of accommodation represents the maximum accommodation of which the eye is capable. Based on the norms of Donders and other reports, Hofstetter[14] provided a formula for the average amplitude of accommodation according to age. We use his formula for determining the *minimum* expected amplitude of accommodation by age: 15 minus 0.25 times the patient's age. For example, a 10-year-old patient should have an amplitude of at least $15 - (0.25 \times 10) = 12.50$ D.

Testing is performed monocularly through the best optical correction of ametropia with a threshold visual acuity target (smallest resolvable at 40 cm). The target is slowly brought closer to the patient as he or she attempts to maintain clarity of the letters. The endpoint is the point at which the letters first become blurred and remain so as testing proceeds. This distance is measured in centimeters from the spectacle plane and converted into dioptric demand for comparison to Hofstetter's formulated age norms. Performance is considered abnormal if the amplitude is more than 2.00 D worse than expected for the patient's age or if there is a significant difference (≥2.00 D) in each eye.

Vergence Skills

Because binocular anomalies affect near-task performance, they have an important role in reading. The demand to coordinate and maintain clear, single binocular vision can be substantial when binocular anomalies are present. In an evaluation and review of the literature, Simons and Grisham[3] came to the conclusion that "exophoria at near and weak fusional vergence reserves are related to reading difficulty." Studies have also found significant correlation between fixation disparity and performance.[15, 16] Correlation between vergence facility and reading difficulty was indicated by Buzzelli.[17] We believe that deficiencies in vergence can contribute to visual symptoms when reading and we, therefore, recommend a sequence of testing to evaluate fusional vergence ability, vergence facility, and fixation disparity.

Relative Vergence

Findings of blur, break, and recovery should be recorded for both positive and negative relative vergence. These findings may be used to help establish the boundaries of the zone of clear, single binocular vision and the application of the criteria of Sheard and Percival in clinical case analysis.[18] General normative data are presented here to assist in the detection of abnormal findings.

With full ametropic lens correction in place, nearpoint testing of positive relative convergence (numbers 16A and 16B of the 21-point examination) is evaluated as follows[19]: A 20/20 equivalent nearpoint target is placed at 40 cm on the nearpoint rod of a phorometer (phoropter) with full illumination. Rotary prisms are set at zero before each eye, and the patient is instructed to try to keep the print clear but to inform the clinician when the letters become blurred, double, or move to one side (i.e., suppression indicated). Base-out prism is then slowly introduced equally to each eye simultaneously until blur, diplopia, or suppression is reported. If blur is reported, the addition of the amount of prism before each eye is the positive relative convergence (16A) finding. Prism continues to be added equally to each eye until diplopia or suppression is reported, which is the base-out break finding. The prism amount is then reduced equally until fusion is reported, which is the recovery finding of 16B. A positive relative convergence blur finding of less than 16^Δ, break of less than 20^Δ, and a recovery of less than 11^Δ is considered abnormal[6] (see Table 9.1).

Evaluating negative relative convergence is similar except that base-in prism is introduced during testing. These measurements are referred to as numbers 17A and 17B of the 21-point examination. A negative relative convergence blur finding of less than 11^Δ, break finding of less than 19^Δ, and a recovery finding of less than 11^Δ is considered abnormal.[6]

Vergence Facility

Vergence facility can be defined as the rate at which positive and negative fusional vergences respond in a given period of time. This ability may have a role in visual performance during reading, and we believe that an evaluation of vergence facility is indicated in cases of RD.

Testing of patients can be performed with an appropriate prism flipper. This is similar to the lens flipper used for accommodative facility testing (see Figure 9.1) except that prisms instead of spherical lenses are used. A target to monitor suppression should be used, such as an SO/V9 Acuity Suppression Slide (see Figure 9.2). Testing is performed at 40 cm with the patient wearing crossed-polarizing filters. The ametropia should be fully corrected while 8^Δ base-out and 8^Δ base-in prisms are alternately introduced with the flipper. Once the clinician has ascertained that the patient is not diplopic or suppressing through either the base-in or base-out demand, the patient is instructed to fixate the letters pointed to by the clinician. The patient is to say each letter aloud when it is seen clearly and singly and is alerted to monitor suppression (disappearance of any letters). Testing continues for 1 minute; the number of fixations called out correctly divided by 2 is the vergence facility rate in cycles per minute (cpm). A facility of less than 5 cpm is the criterion for inadequate performance.[6]

Vergence Accuracy

Accuracy of the vergence system can be evaluated through assessment of fixation disparity. Fixation disparity has been defined as "a small misalignment of the two eyes during binocular fusion."[20] The presence of a horizontal fixation disparity at near may affect reading performance.[15, 16] Sheedy's Disparometer (Vision Analysis, Walnut Creek, CA) is useful for fine measurement of fixation disparity (y intercept), associated phoria (the amount of prism necessary to eliminate the fixation disparity, x intercept), and generation of a fixation disparity curve (Figure 9.3). The Wesson Fixation Disparity Card (Vision Extension of the Optometric Extension Program Foundation, Inc., Santa Ana, CA) (Figure 9.4) is a useful clinical tool for the screening of fixation disparity; it can also be used to determine the x intercept and estimate the y intercept and shape of the curve.[21] Commercially available devices and their clinical utility are reviewed by Brownlee and Goss.[22]

Numerous studies have related asthenopic symptoms at nearpoint with fixation disparity characteristics.[23–27] We recommend determination of the fixation disparity curve at nearpoint when there is a history of RD.

Both the Disparometer and the Wesson Card have test marks on the target that are seen separately through polarizing filters; the standard setup results in the upper test mark seen by the right eye and the lower mark seen by the left eye. Both instruments have a fusion lock. The Disparometer fusion stimulus is a circle that subtends 1.5

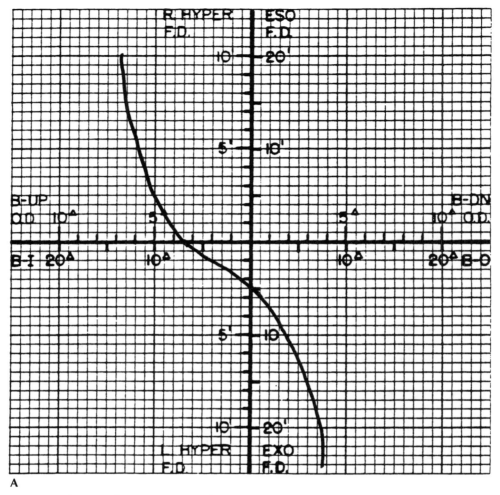

FIGURE 9.3 *Fixation disparity curves showing y intercept, x intercept, and shape of the forced-vergence fixation disparity curve. A. Abnormal curve with steep slope. B. Normal curve with flat slope.*

degrees, and the Wesson Card has a 1-cm square black border. With no prism in place (and the target mark set at zero with the Disparometer), the patient reports that the test marks are aligned or that the upper mark is off to the right or left of the lower mark. If the marks are reported as misaligned, a fixation disparity is present; the lower mark to the left of the upper mark indicates eso fixation disparity, the lower mark to the right of the upper mark indicates exo fixation disparity. The amount of fixation disparity is determined by sequentially presenting different pairs of vernier lines with increasing misalignment within the fusion circle until the lines appear aligned to the patient.[20] The amount of fixation disparity in minutes of arc can then be read from the examiner's side of the instrument. The amount of fix-

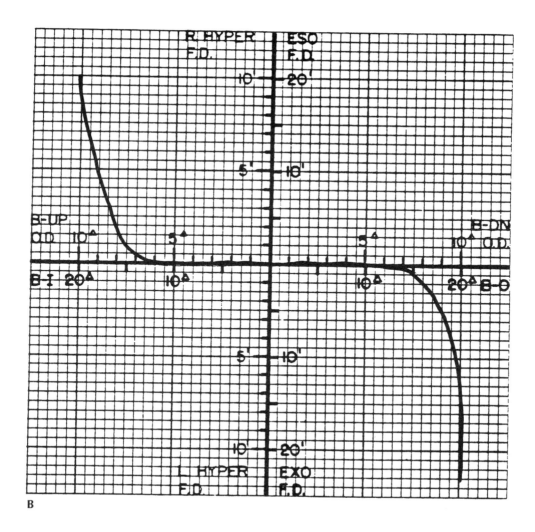

B

ation disparity is shown on the Wesson Card in minutes of arc by comparing the colored line the lower arrow is pointing to with the table of values on the face of the card.[21]

Visual-Perceptual-Motor Skills

As discussed in Chapter 6, significant correlation between test results for VPM development and reading readiness has been found for children in kindergarten and the early primary grades.[28] VPM function, therefore, plays an important role based on the written symbolic and representational demands in our highly literate society. For example, reading requires the individual to interpret the shapes and directional orientations of the alphabet and number system. Testing and analysis of VPM functions have been presented

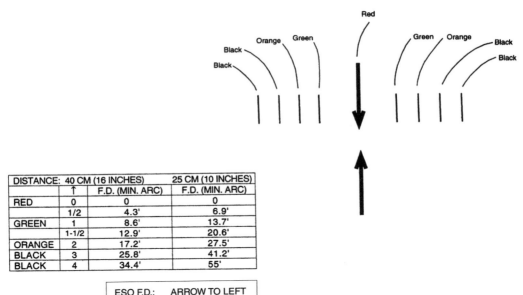

DISTANCE:	40 CM (16 INCHES)		25 CM (10 INCHES)
	↑	F.D. (MIN. ARC)	F.D. (MIN. ARC)
RED	0	0	0
	1/2	4.3'	6.9'
GREEN	1	8.6'	13.7'
	1-1/2	12.9'	20.6'
ORANGE	2	17.2'	27.5'
BLACK	3	25.8'	41.2'
BLACK	4	34.4'	55'

ESO F.D.:	ARROW TO LEFT
EXO F.D.:	ARROW TO RIGHT

FIGURE 9.4   *Wesson Fixation Disparity Card.*

numerous times in the literature[29–31]; but nomenclature for this type of testing has changed more than the tests themselves. It is currently in vogue to refer to these VPM functions (Table 9.2) as visual information–processing skills.

Scoring and interpretation of perceptual tests usually requires conversion of a raw score into a relative measure, referred to as a derived score.[30, 32, 33] Derived scores (e.g., scaled score, standard score, percentile rank) allow direct comparison of performance to a normative sample and to performance on other tests. Performance is generally considered weak if test results are more than half of one standard deviation below the norm.[32] Some tests convert raw scores to developmental norms (age or grade equivalents) based on the mean or median raw score obtained on a test by a specific age group or grade level.[32] We consider performance weak if the score yields an age equivalent more than 1 year below chronologic age or a grade equivalent more than 1 year below grade placement. It is important to remember, however, that observations of performance and case history results are equally influential in determining the diagnosis.[30]

Bilateral Integration

Several tests evaluate the visual-spatial skill of bilateral integration. The bilateral integration test we prefer and routinely administer is the *chalkboard circles test*. We use the test to assess body knowledge and con-

TABLE 9.2   Visual-Perceptual-Motor Skills and Testing Methods

Function	Testing Procedure
Bilateral integration	Chalkboard circles
Laterality	Piaget left-right awareness
Directionality	Piaget left-right awareness
Directionality for numbers and letters	Gardner Reversals Frequency Test (recognition)
Visual discrimination	Test of Visual Perceptual Skills
Visual memory	Test of Visual Perceptual Skills
Visual-spatial relationships	Test of Visual Perceptual Skills
Visual form constancy	Test of Visual Perceptual Skills
Visual sequential memory	Test of Visual Perceptual Skills
Visual figure-ground	Test of Visual Perceptual Skills
Visual closure	Test of Visual Perceptual Skills
Visual-motor integration	Beery Test of Visual-Motor Integration
Sentence copy skill	Wold Sentence Copy Test
Auditory-visual integration	Auditory-Visual Integration Test
Auditory discrimination	Test of Auditory-Perceptual Skills

trol, which is the relative integrity of the invariant.[29] The test requires a large chalkboard and two pieces of chalk. The patient is instructed to face the center of the chalkboard with a piece of chalk in each hand while the examiner demonstrates the task in the air by taking each of the patient's arms and simulating the circles. Each circle should have a diameter of approximately 1 ft (Figure 9.5). The test has two parts, production of symmetric circles and of reciprocal circles. In the symmetric circles portion, one hand makes a clockwise circle while the other hand makes a counterclockwise circle. At least five revolutions should be attempted. Reciprocal circles are then attempted; both hands make either clockwise or counterclockwise circular movements. The patient is instructed to keep repeating the circles without stopping, and without the circles touching each other, until the examiner says "stop." At least five revolutions should be performed. When the patient has attempted five revolutions of reciprocal circles, he is asked to stop and reverse the direction of both circles for five revolutions.

The patient's performance is compared with characteristic performance of other patients of the same age[29] to determine the age level of the child's performance. More than 1 year below age-expected performance is considered inadequate.

Laterality and Directionality

Laterality and directionality skills are important to the organization of external visual space and understanding of directional concepts.[30] *Laterality* refers to the knowledge of one's own right and left. *Directionality* is the understanding of right and left directions in exter-

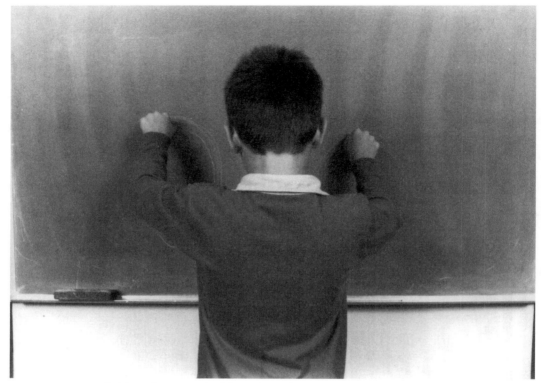

FIGURE 9.5 *A child performing chalkboard circles.*

nal space. These spatial skills are important in many aspects of learning and probably have specific relevance to reading in the development of language symbol recognition. Development of laterality and directionality abilities follows a well-documented maturational sequence.[29–31, 34–37] We routinely administer the Piaget test of left-right awareness to evaluate laterality and directionality. This test is not commercially available, but the instruction set is provided in Table 9.3A.[30, 31, 34]

The Piaget test of left-right awareness has five sections, each of which contains questions that probe the patient's laterality and directionality knowledge. Every question in each section must be answered correctly for the patient to pass that section. Age-equivalent performance is determined by the sections the patient was able to pass. Note that, developmentally, section C is normally mastered before section B (Table 9.3B). Performance that is more than 1 year below age-expected performance is considered inadequate.

Directionality for Numbers and Letters

Application of directionality concepts to language symbols is integral to understanding the correct orientation of numbers and letters. There

TABLE 9.3A   Directions for the Piaget Test of Left-Right Awareness

Test questions
A. Show me your right hand. Show me your left leg.
    Touch your left ear. Raise your right hand.
    Show me your right leg.
    Show me your left hand.
    Point to your right eye.
B. (Sit opposite the child.)
    Show me my right hand.
    Now show me my left hand.
    Show me my right leg.
    Now my left leg.
C. (Place a coin on the table left of a pencil in relation to the child.)
    Is the pencil to the right or to the left?
    And the penny, is it to the right or to the left?
    (Have the child go around to the opposite side of the table.)
    Is the pencil to the right or to the left?
    And the penny, is it to the right or to the left?
D. (Sit opposite the child with a coin in your right hand and a bracelet or watch on your left
        arm.)
    You see this penny: Have I got it in my right hand or in the left?
    And the bracelet: Is it on my right arm or my left?
E. (Place three objects in front of the child: a pencil to the left, a key in the middle, and a coin to
        the right.)
    Is the pencil to the left or to the right of the key?
    Is the pencil to the left or to the right of the penny?
    Is the key to the left or to the right of the penny?
    Is the key to the left or to the right of the pencil?
    Is the penny to the left or to the right of the pencil?
    Is the penny to the left or to the right of the key?

TABLE 9.3B   Norms for the Piaget Test of Left-Right Awareness

Age	Items Passed by 75% of Age Group
5	A
6	A
7	A, C
8	A, B, C, D
9	A, B, C, D
10	A, B, C, D
11	A, B, C, D, E

are two principal methods to assess directionality abilities: (1) evaluating the patient's ability to write letters and numbers and (2) examining the patient's ability to judge which numbers and letters in an array are either reversed or oriented correctly. We use two subtests of the Gardner Reversals Frequency Test (Creative Therapeutics, Cresskill, NJ) to evaluate these abilities.[38]

The execution subtest requires the child to write letters and numbers in the correct orientation on a test form as they are dictated. The child writes the numbers with a pencil as each one is dictated, in the following order: 2, 5, 6, 3, 9, 4, 7. The child is then instructed to print lowercase letters as each one is dictated. The letters are dictated in the following order: h, c, q, f, j, b, k, s, r, d, y, p, t, z, g, a, e. The testing environment should be such that materials with printing cannot be seen by the patient. The patient (usually a child but in some cases an adult) is allowed to erase and rewrite any of the symbols. This subtest is scored by the number and type of errors made. If a letter is reversed, it is scored as a reversal error; if the child cannot remember a letter or writes the wrong letter, it is scored as an unknown error. These types of errors are scored separately, and the test manual contains tables that allow conversion of the raw scores of unknown and reversal errors into percentile rank scores by age. These tables are also divided by gender.

The recognition subtest of the Gardner Reversals Frequency Test requires the child to determine which letters and numbers in an array are reversed and which are correctly oriented. There are six rows of symbols, and the task gets progressively difficult with each row (Figure 9.6). The child is instructed to cross out each letter and number that appears to be backward; erasing is allowed. There is no time limit for this test. The subtest is scored by the number of errors made. An error is either a reversed symbol that was not crossed out or a symbol in the correct orientation that was crossed out. The total number of errors made is the raw score. There are scoring tables in the test manual to convert the raw score into a percentile rank score by age.

Motor-Free Visual Perception

To evaluate specific subskills integral to the analysis of visual information, we use the test of visual perceptual skills (TVPS).[39] The TVPS is designed for ages 4–13, but an adult version is also available. The test has seven subtest areas: visual discrimination, visual memory, visual-spatial relationships, visual figure-ground, visual sequential memory, visual form constancy, and visual closure. These visual skills most likely contribute to the ability to recognize language symbols and eventually to the recognition of words as visual gestalts. There is a practice plate (plate A) and 16 test plates in each subtest. The patient should answer plate A correctly before proceeding with the test items. The instructions need to be restated and the correct answer pointed out before proceeding if the response on plate A is incorrect. If there are five possible answers to choose from, testing on the subtest is stopped when the patient has missed four of five consecutive test items. Similarly, if there are four possible answers to choose from, testing on the subtest is stopped when the patient has missed three of four consecutive test items.

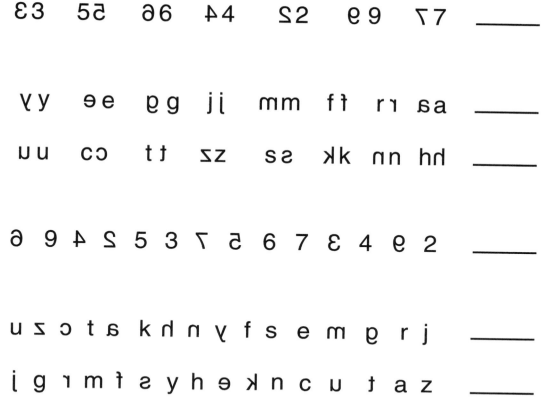

FIGURE 9.6 *Recognition testing of letter and number reversals in the Gardner Reversals Frequency Test. (Redrawn from RA Gardner. The Objective Diagnosis of Minimal Brain Dysfunction. Cresskill, NJ: Creative Therapeutics, 1979.)*

Visual Discrimination

The visual discrimination subtest requires the patient to examine a form and pick the form from an array of similar shapes containing one form that is exactly the same (Figure 9.7).

Visual Memory

A similar task is required in the visual memory subtest, but the original form is presented for 5 seconds on a separate page from the possible answers; then the patient is asked to remember the original form when selecting an answer.

Visual Sequential Memory

Visual sequential memory is evaluated in the same manner as visual memory, but there is more than one form on the original plate. When selecting the answer for this subtest, the forms must be remembered

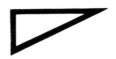

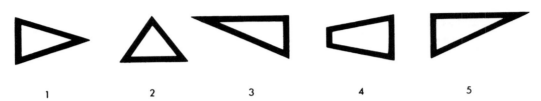

| 1 | 2 | 3 | 4 | 5 |

FIGURE 9.7 *The visual discrimination subtest of the Test of Visual Perceptual Skills. (Reprinted by permission of MF Gardner. Test of Visual Perceptual Skills. Burlingame, CA: Psychological and Educational Publications, 1988.)*

in the proper order. The patient is allowed progressively more time to view and remember the original plate as the number of forms to be remembered increases. The times allowed for viewing the original plates are as follows: 5 seconds for 2–3 forms, 9 seconds for 3–5 forms, 12 seconds for 6–7 forms, and 14 seconds for 8–9 forms.

Visual-Spatial Relationships

For the visual-spatial relationships subtest, the patient is asked to pick the one form that is different from the others (Figure 9.8).

Visual Figure-Ground

To evaluate visual figure-ground skills, the patient is asked to examine a form and find this form hidden in other patterns (Figure 9.9).

Visual Form Constancy

The visual form constancy subtest is similar to the visual figure-ground test, but the hidden form may be larger, smaller, darker, or turned on its side.

Visual Closure

Visual closure requires the patient to look at the form on top and find the incomplete form in the array below that would look exactly like the top form if all of the lines were connected (Figure 9.10).

Each subtest is scored individually using the TVPS scoring manual to convert raw scores into percentile ranks by age.

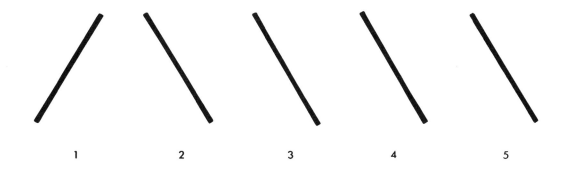

1   2   3   4   5

FIGURE 9.8 *The visual-spatial relationships subtest of the Test of Visual Perceptual Skills. (Reprinted by permission of MF Gardner. Test of Visual Perceptual Skills. Burlingame, CA: Psychological and Educational Publications, 1988.)*

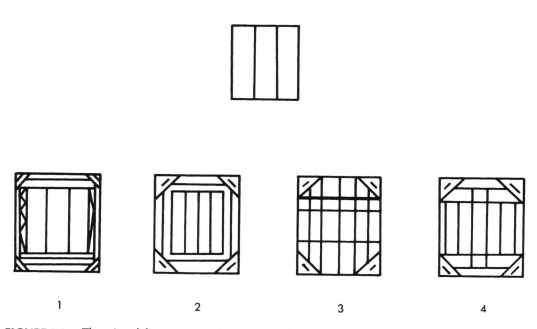

1   2   3   4

FIGURE 9.9 *The visual figure-ground subtest of the Test of Visual Perceptual Skills. (Reprinted by permission of MF Gardner. Test of Visual Perceptual Skills. Burlingame, CA: Psychological and Educational Publications, 1988.)*

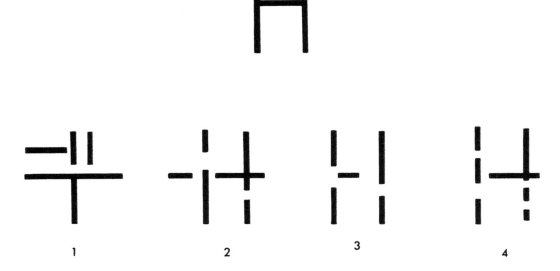

FIGURE 9.10   *The visual closure subtest of the Test of Visual Perceptual Skills. (Reprinted by permission of MF Gardner. Test of Visual Perceptual Skills. Burlingame, CA: Psychological and Educational Publications, 1988.)*

Visual-Motor Integration

Visual-motor integration is commonly referred to as eye-hand coordination, but it also involves the ability to guide motor movements along with visual analysis skills. We use the revised Developmental Test of Visual Motor Integration[40] to evaluate this perceptual area. This test was normed for ages 3–15 years and requires the patient to copy a sequence of forms as accurately as possible (Figure 9.11). The patient is not allowed to trace the forms, erase any parts, or make sketchy lines when copying the forms. The test presents forms in progressively higher levels of developmental difficulty, and the test should be stopped when the patient has been unsuccessful in copying three consecutive forms.

Scoring the test involves the use of specific grading criteria for each individual form. These criteria are supplied in the test manual, and failure to meet all criteria for a given form constitutes a score of zero points for that particular form. Scoring is weighted according to level of difficulty, and each form is worth 1–4 points (provided in the scoring manual) if copied within the given criteria, depending on the developmental demand of the form. The raw score is the total number of points achieved until the test was terminated, and this score can be converted into a percentile rank score by age using the tables provided in the test manual.

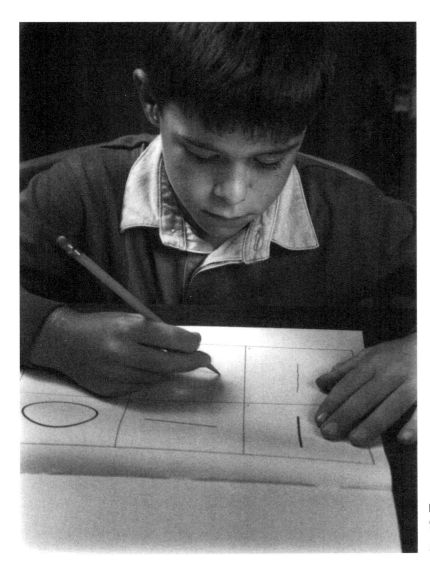

FIGURE 9.11 *A child performing the Test of Visual-Motor Integration.*

Sentence Copy Skills

The Wold Sentence Copy Test[41, 42] is used to evaluate visual-motor integration skill on a language-based task. This test requires the patient to copy a long sentence onto lines provided below (Figure 9.12). The patient is asked to copy the sentence as quickly and as accurately as possible. The patient may write in cursive or print, but the writing should be neat and easy to read.

This test is scored by taking the number of symbols copied (110 if performed accurately) multiplied by 60, and dividing this calculated number by the time (in seconds) taken to complete the task. This gives a score in letters copied per minute. This score can be compared to grade-equivalent performance using Table 9.4.

Four men and a jolly boy came out of the black and pink house quickly to see the bright violet sun, but the sun was hidden behind a cloud.

_____

_____

_____

_____

_____

_____

FIGURE 9.12 *The Wold Sentence Copy Test. (Redrawn from RM Wold. Screening Tests to Be Used by the Classroom Teacher. Novato, CA: Academic Therapy Publications, 1970;4–5.)*

TABLE 9.4   Scoring Criteria for the Wold Sentence Copy Test

Grade	Rate of Handwriting (Letters/Min)
2	39.7
3	42.0
4	45.8
5	50.5
6	54.5
7	53.9
8	62.8

Auditory-Perceptual Skills

Two areas of auditory-perceptual skills are discussed. Problems with these skills may result in RD.

Auditory-Visual Integration

Auditory-visual integration is the ability to match what is heard with what is seen. This matching of auditory stimuli with visual stimuli is exemplified in the interpretation of Morse code. In reading, we attempt to match visual stimuli (letters, syllables, and words) with the sounds they represent. We use the auditory-visual integration test, originally described by Birch and Belmont[43–45] to evaluate this skill. The test is currently available through Vision Extension of the Optometric Extension Program Foundation in an expanded format with normative data.[46]

The test uses dot patterns with various spacings printed on cards that represent the previously presented auditory stimuli. The clinician taps one of three patterns on a card, and the patient is then shown the card

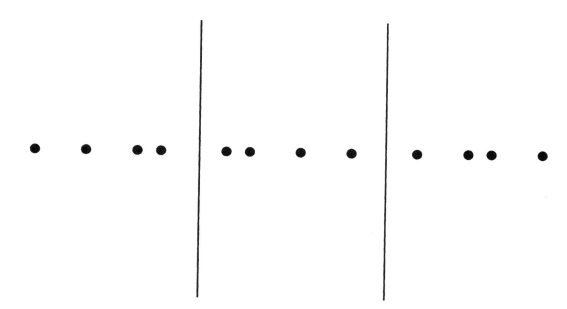

FIGURE 9.13   *An item on the Auditory-Visual Integration Test. (Redrawn from HG Birch, L Belmont. Auditory-Visual Integration Test. Santa Ana, CA: Optometric Extension Program Foundation, 1995.)*

and asked which visual pattern had been produced auditorily. There are three demonstration cards and 20 test cards; only the first 10 are used for children 10 years old or younger; all 20 are used for patients over 10 years old (Figure 9.13). The demonstration cards have specific instructions that sequentially introduce the patient to the task. Demonstration card A is shown to the patient, and the examiner taps out each of the three dot patterns to familiarize the patient with how the spacing and dot series should sound. The examiner then shows the patient demonstration card B and taps out the selected pattern, asking the patient to point to the pattern that was tapped. For demonstration card C, the selected pattern is tapped before the card is shown to the patient for determination of which pattern was tapped; this is how the test cards are presented for subsequent testing. It is recommended that the hand used for tapping the patterns be out of view of the patient. The raw score for this test is the number of correct responses given. Tables are provided in the testing manual to determine whether performance is within an expected age level.

Auditory Discrimination

We believe testing of auditory discrimination skills should be included in cases of RD. Auditory discrimination is the ability to discern subtle differences between stimuli presented solely in an auditory fashion. This auditory processing skill is crucial to reading and cognitive development because it enables the child to discriminate between words with phonemically similar consonants, cognates, or vowel differences. Although poor readers would be expected to perform below their age level on auditory discrimination tests, this relationship is inconclusive.[47] According to Wepman,[48] auditory discrimination for words is an ability that gradually increases with age until about the age of 9. We use the auditory discrimination subtest of the Test of Auditory-Perceptual Skills[49] to evaluate this ability. It is important to bear in mind that this test has an inherent component of auditory memory, which may affect the interpretation of results.

The patient must be able to understand and apply the concept of "same versus different" to respond appropriately on this test. The clinician says two words (one to two syllables long), and the patient is asked to determine if the paired words were the same or different. Several practice examples should be given before proceeding to the test itself. The patient listens to the words *net* and *neck*, for example, and responds with "same" or "different." The patient should face away from the examiner while the test word pairs are slowly (interval of 1–2 seconds between words) enunciated in a soft, audible tone close to the back of the patient's head. It is important that the pronunciation of both the clinician and patient be basically the same to prevent potential problems with reliability and validity. For example, some Southerners may pronounce *card* as *cod* and some Bostonians may say *cad*.

The test consists of 50 word pairs, 36 of which are different and 14 that are identical. The patient's response to each of the word pairs is recorded and used in scoring the test. The 14 identical word pairs are used to determine the validity of the test administration; the 36 different word pairs provide the raw score used to determine the patient's auditory discrimination ability. Scoring tables based on age-expected performance are provided in the test manual, as are conversion tables for percentile ranks.[49]

Summary

We recommend a thorough evaluation of VSE and VPM skills when there is a history of reading difficulties. Evaluation of vision efficiency skills should include testing of oculomotor, accommodative, and binocular skills. Evaluation of VPM skills should include testing for skills of bilateral integration, laterality, directionality, directionality for letters and numbers, motor-free visual perception, visual-motor integration, sentence copying, and auditory perception. Deficiencies in these skills can either contribute to or be the single cause of RD. Vision therapy is effective to improve vision efficiency and VPM abilities (pertinent and effective vision therapy procedures are presented in Chapter 11).

References

1. Special report: the efficacy of optometric vision therapy. The 1986/87 Future of Visual Development/Performance Task Force. J Am Optom Assoc 1988;59:95–105.
2. Grisham JD, Simons HD. Refractive error and the reading process: a literature analysis. J Am Optom Assoc 1986;57:44–55.
3. Simons HD, Grisham JD. Binocular anomalies and reading problems. J Am Optom Assoc 1987;58:578–87.
4. Simons HD, Gassler PA. Vision anomalies and reading skill: a meta-analysis of the literature. Am J Optom Physiol Opt 1988;65:893–904.
5. Harris AJ. How many kinds of reading disabilities are there? J Learn Disabil 1982;15:456–60.
6. Griffin JR, Grisham JD. Binocular Anomalies: Diagnosis and Vision Therapy (3rd ed). Boston: Butterworth-Heinemann, 1995.
7. Richman JE, Garcia RP. Developmental Eye Movement Test (DEM). South Bend, IN: Bernell Corp., 1987.
8. Hoffman LG, Rouse MW. Referral recommendations for binocular function and/or developmental perceptual deficiencies. J Am Optom Assoc 1980;51:119–25.
9. Hennessey D, Iosue RA, Rouse MW. Relation of symptoms to accommodative infacility of school-aged children. Am J Optom Physiol Opt 1984;61:177–83.
10. Zellers JA, Alpert TL, Rouse MW. A review of the literature and a normative study of accommodative facility. J Am Optom Assoc 1984;55:31–7.
11. Haynes HM. Clinical observations with dynamic retinoscopy. Optom Weekly 1960;51:2243–6, 2306–9.
12. Rouse MW, London R, Allen DC. An evaluation of the monocular estimate method of dynamic retinoscopy. Am J Optom Physiol Opt 1982;59:234–9.
13. Rouse MW, Hutter RF, Shiftlett R. A normative study of accommodative lag in elementary school children. Am J Optom Physiol Opt 1984;61:693–7.
14. Cline D, Hofstetter HW, Griffin JR (eds). Dictionary of Visual Science (4th ed). Radnor, PA: Chilton, 1989;277.
15. Silbiger F, Woolf D. Fixation disparity and reading achievement at the college level. Am J Optom Arch Am Acad Optom 1968;45:734–42.
16. O'Grady J. The relationship between vision and educational performance: a study of year 2 children in Tasmania. Aust J Optom 1984;67:126–40.
17. Buzzelli AR. Stereopsis, accommodative and vergence facility: do they relate to dyslexia? Optom Vis Sci 1991;68:842–6.
18. Goss DA. Ocular Accommodation, Convergence, and Fixation Disparity: A Manual of Clinical Analysis. Boston: Butterworth, 1986;23–4, 47–51, 53–56.
19. Hendrickson H. The Behavioral Optometry Approach to Lens Prescribing. Duncan, OK: Optometric Extension Program, 1980;13–4.
20. Sheedy JE. Actual measurement of fixation disparity and its use in diagnosis and treatment. J Am Optom Assoc 1980;51:1079–84.
21. Wesson MD, Koenig R. A new clinical method for direct measurement of fixation disparity. South J Optom 1983;1:48–52.

22. Brownlee GA, Goss DA. Comparisons of commercially available devices for the measurement of fixation disparity and associated phorias. J Am Optom Assoc 1988;59:451–60.

23. Arner RS, Berger SI, Braverman G, et al. The clinical significance of the effect of vergence on fixation disparity: a preliminary investigation. Am J Optom Arch Am Acad Optom 1956;33:399–409.

24. Sheedy JE, Saladin JJ. Exophoria at near in presbyopia. Am J Optom Physiol Optics 1975;52:474–81.

25. Sheedy JE, Saladin JJ. Phoria, vergence, and fixation disparity in oculomotor problems. Am J Optom Physiol Optics 1977;54:474–8.

26. Sheedy JE, Saladin JJ. Association of symptoms with measures of oculomotor deficiencies. Am J Optom Physiol Optics 1978;55:670–6.

27. Sheedy JE. Fixation disparity analysis of oculomotor imbalance. Am J Optom Physiol Optics 1980;57:632–9.

28. Solan HA, Mozlin R. The correlations of perceptual-motor maturation to readiness and reading in kindergarten and the primary grades. J Am Optom Assoc 1986;57:28–35.

29. Suchoff IB. Visual-Spatial Development in the Child: An Optometric Theoretical and Clinical Approach. New York: SUNY College of Optometry, 1973.

30. Schieman MM, Rouse MW. Optometric Management of Learning-Related Vision Problems. St. Louis: Mosby, 1994.

31. Groffman S, Solan HA. Developmental and Perceptual Assessment of Learning-Disabled Children: Theoretical Concepts and Diagnostic Testing. Santa Ana, CA: Optometric Extension Program, 1994.

32. Solan HA, Suchoff IB. Test and Measurements for Behavioral Optometrists. Santa Ana, CA: Optometric Extension Program, 1991.

33. Anastasi A. Psychological Testing (6th ed). New York: Macmillan, 1988.

34. Piaget J. Judgment and Reasoning in the Child. London: Routledge & Kegan Paul, 1928;96–134.

35. Laurendeau M, Pinard A. The Development of the Concept of Space in the Child. New York: International Universities Press, 1970;278–309.

36. Ilg FL, Ames LB. School Readiness: Behavior Tests Used at the Gesell Institute. New York: Harper & Row, 1972;159–89.

37. Kuczaj SA, Maratsos MP. On the acquisition of front, back and side. Child Dev 1975;46:202–10.

38. Gardner RA. The Objective Diagnosis of Minimal Brain Dysfunction. Cresskill, NJ: Creative Therapeutics, 1979.

39. Gardner MF. Test of Visual Perceptual Skills. Burlingame, CA: Psychological and Educational Publications, 1988.

40. Beery KE, Buktenica NA. Developmental Test of Visual-Motor Integration (3rd rev). Columbus, OH: Modern Curriculum Press, 1989.

41. Wold RM. Screening Tests to Be Used by the Classroom Teacher. Novato, CA: Academic Therapy Publications, 1970;4–5.

42. Griffin J. Comparison of two sentence copy tests. Optom Monthly 1984;74:410–6.

43. Birch HG, Belmont L. Auditory-visual integration, intelligence and reading ability in school children. Percept Mot Skills 1965;20:295–305.

44. Birch HG, Belmont L. Auditory-visual integration in normal and retarded readers. Am J Orthopsychiatry 1964;34:852–61.

45. Birch HG, Belmont L. Auditory-visual integration in brain-damaged and normal children. Dev Med Child Neurol 1965;7:135–44.
46. Birch HG, Belmont L. Auditory-Visual Integration Test. Santa Ana, CA: Optometric Extension Program Foundation, 1995.
47. Dystra R. Auditory discrimination abilities and beginning reading achievement. Reading Res Q 1966;1:5–34.
48. Wepman JM. Auditory discrimination: its role in language comprehension, formulation and use. Pediatr Clin North Am 1968;15:721–7.
49. Gardner MF. Test of Auditory-Perceptual Skills. Burlingame, CA: Psychological and Educational Publications, 1985.

10 **Testing of Dyslexia**

Before dyslexia can be diagnosed, general contributory causes of reading dysfunction (RD) must be ruled out, such as low intelligence, educational deprivation, and vision problems (see Chapter 1). These exclusionary and indirect factors that can cause *general* RD must be ruled out to confirm direct testing results. The two direct tests for dyslexia are the Boder Test of Reading and Spelling Patterns[1] and the Dyslexia Determination Test (DDT).[2] We consider only the DDT in this text, for several reasons. Unlike the DDT, the eidetic encoding challenge of the Boder test uses both phonetically regular and irregular words as task stimuli and makes no provision for testing of dysnemkinetic dyslexia. The DDT was the first formal test for direct diagnosis of dyslexia (1981) made available to practitioners, it is the most widely

Table 10.1 Various Tests, Screeners, and Therapy Material for Dyslexia

Name	Age or Grade	Publisher
Dyslexia Determination Test (DDT)[2]	Grades 2–12	IMED
Boder Test of Reading and Spelling Patterns[1]	Grades 2–12	GS
Spanish Screening Version of DDT[4]	Grades 2–12	IMED
French Screening Version of DDT[5]	Grades 2–12	RPTC
The Dyslexia Screener (TDS)[6]	Grades 2–9	RPTC
Adult Dyslexia Test (ADT)[7]	≥18 years	RPTC
Dyslexia Screener for First-graders (DSF)[8]	Grade 1	RPTC
Predyslexia Letter Coding Test (PLCT)[9]	Kindergarten	RPTC
Home Dyslexia Screening Test (HDST)[10]	Grades 2–9	CTC
Therapy in Dyslexia and Reading Problems[3]	All ages	IMED

IMED = Instructional Materials and Equipment Distributors, Los Angeles, CA; GS = Grune & Stratton, New York (also distributed by Academic Therapy Publishers, Novato, CA); RPTC = Reading and Perception Therapy Center, Culver City, CA; CTC = Christenson Therapy Center, Hudson, WI.

used and easily administered test, and it is available in English, Spanish, and French. Other tests compatible with the DDT are the Predyslexia Letter Coding Test (PLCT) for kindergartners, Dyslexia Screener for First-graders (DSF), the Adult Dyslexia Test (ADT), and The Dyslexia Screener (TDS), a quick, easy-to-administer, shortened version of the DDT. Finally, a therapy book[3] is available for dyslexia that is an extension of the DDT (Table 10.1). Once the clinician masters administration, interpretation, and evaluation of the DDT, the other similar tests are easy to learn and administer. (Note that the authors of this text are some of the coauthors of the DDT, PLCT, DSF, ADT, TDS, or tests in other languages. Research and clinical experience led to development of these assessment tools.)

Characteristics of a Dyslexia Test

The DDT is composed of three parts: (1) testing for reversals of numbers and letters, for the diagnosis of dysnemkinetic dyslexia; (2) testing of eidetic coding of whole words, for the diagnosis of dyseidetic dyslexia; and (3) testing of phonetic coding for syllabication, for the diagnosis of dysphonetic dyslexia. In the first part of the test, the patient prints the numbers 1–10 and then prints (in noncursive writing) the alphabet in upper- and lowercase letters. Reversal errors are totaled and the results evaluated. The second part of the test involves decoding words selected by ascending grade levels. The odd-numbered words are phonetically irregular; the even-numbered words are phonetically regular (i.e., spelled fairly faithfully the way the words sound). Words are checked off as decoded eidetically (E column) if they have been correctly pronounced (in the patient's variation of accent and dialect) within 2 seconds of viewing time. Words have been decoded phonetically (P column) if the time required for a correct response was more than 2 seconds (10-second maximum allowed). Unknown words are tallied in the U column. The mode of decoding (see Chapter 3) is evaluated according to the instruction manual of the DDT. Basically, poor eidetic decoding (look-say skills) is indicated if the eidetic decoding level is below the grade placement. This type of patient is also usually able to decode many more words on a phonetic basis, especially the even-numbered, phonetically regular words. Conversely, poor phonetic decoding is indicated if the eidetic decoding level is high compared to phonetic decoding ability. In such cases, the patient is able to decode relatively few words on a phonetic basis, even when sufficient time is allowed (poor word-attack skills).

The third part of the DDT consists of encoding tasks, wherein the patient must spell words from dictation. In the eidetic encoding challenge, the patient attempts to spell words at his or her decoding level and downward to lower levels until the basal (10 odd-numbered E-column words) is reached. These dictated words are flash known (identified in ≤2 seconds) and have phonetically irregular spelling (e.g., *listen* and *does*, which are odd numbered, as opposed to phonetically regular words, such as *just* and *ask*, which are even numbered). In the phonetic encoding challenge, the patient tries to spell phonetic equivalents of unknown words at and beyond his or her decoding level. It does not matter whether the unknown word (i.e., a word the patient is unable to decode either on an eidetic or phonetic basis) to be dictated is odd or even numbered. The purpose here is to determine whether the patient can write a good phonetic equivalent of a word on hearing it. For example, if the patient is unable to decode the word *listen*; it is considered an unknown word. When the clinician dictates that word and the patient writes *lisen* (or *lisun, lesin, lesun, lesen,* or *lisin)*, the response is considered correct. Any reasonable, phonetically good equivalent is allowed.

The DDT has two alternate decoding forms (A and B) for test and retest purposes. The format is the same, but the word lists are different. Complete instructions are provided in the DDT testing kit.

Dyseidesia

Figure 10.1 shows the decoding part of the DDT results of an 11-year-old in the fifth grade who is reading at the second-grade level (Case 1).

Decoding

In this example, the patient's eidetic decoding level is at the second grade, as determined by the 50% psychometric method (the highest grade at which the patient has half or more correct responses). The

Checklist Sheet

Date _____

DDT Decoding Patterns for FORM A
RECORDING PAGE

Examinee's
Name _____

Birth
Date _____ Yrs. _11_ Mos. _4_

AGE

Grade
Placement _5 Th_

Odd Numbered Words — Non Phonetic
Even Numbered Words — Phonetic

p-primer	E	P	U		primer	E	P	U		1st	E	P	U		2nd	E	P	U
1 green					1 are	✓			(x)	1 money	✓			(x)	1 does	✓		
2 an					2 yes	✓				2 him		✓			2 ask		✓	
3 look					3 ready	✓			(x)	3 call	✓				3 listen			(x)
4 go					4 did	✓				4 if	✓				4 just		✓	
5 mother					5 lock	✓			(x)	5 guess	✓			(x)	5 uncle	✓		
6 no					6 up	✓				6 fast		✓			6 sled	✓		
7 said					7 black	✓			(x)	7 funny	✓			(x)	7 city	✓		
8 stop				8	8 on	✓				8 we	✓				8 step	✓		
9 ball				(x)	9 came	✓			(x)	9 here	✓			(x)	9 rolled	✓		
10 in					10 it	✓				10 with	✓				10 wet	✓		
Totals					Totals	10	0	0		Totals	8	2	0		Totals	6	3	1

3rd	E	P	U		4th	E	P	U		5th	E	P	U		6th	E	P	U
1 business		✓			1 delight		✓			1 height					1 badge			
2 lamp	✓				2 human	✓				2 invent					2 abandon			
3 believe		✓			3 familiar		✓			3 doubt					3 conceited			
4 jump	✓				4 pupils		✓			4 planted					4 melting			
5 heavy		✓			5 soared		✓			5 position					5 foreign			
6 path	✓				6 trunk	✓				6 grand					6 album			
7 laugh	✓				7 rough		✓			7 contagious					7 knapsack			
8 drink	✓				8 whisk	✓				8 handed					8 varnish			
9 should		✓			9 glisten		✓			9 vowed					9 decisions			
10 dish		✓			10 prison		✓			10 ambush					10 shifted			
Totals	1	4	5		Totals	0	4	6		Totals					Totals	—	—	—

7—8	E	P	U		9—12	E	P	U		College	E	P	U		Column Designations
1 coolie					1 heinous					1 homologous					
2 edit					2 minus					2 emigrant					"E" — Flash Known
3 graciously					3 graduation					3 homeopathy					(Eidetic)
4 blunt					4 detested					4 subabdominal					"P" — Untimed Known
5 tomorrow					5 pollute					5 rheostat					(Phonetic)
6 abhor					6 digit					6 admonish					"U" — Unknown Words
7 trudge					7 snuggle					7 demagogue					
8 devoted					8 prevalent					8 demented					
9 aeronautic					9 exonerate					9 euphony					
10 abolish					10 bonus					10 minuet					
Totals	—	—	—		Totals	—	—	—		Totals	—	—	—		

Results of Decoding — FORM A

Highest grade level of sight word recognition (50% Flash Known) _____ 2nd _____
Number of Flash-Known words at DDT Grade Level _____ 6 _____

Decoding Mode:

Relatively more phonetic ☑︎   Relatively more eidetic ☐   Relatively equal ☐

Comments: _____
_____
_____
_____

Examiner: _____   Date: _____

FIGURE 10.1   *Decoding results in 11-year-old in fifth grade (Case 1).*

patient was able to decode 100% (10 of 10) words at the primer level
(beginning of the first grade). (*Primer* is usually pronounced
preh'muhr.) At the first-grade level, the patient decoded 80% of the E
words; at the second-grade level, the patient decoded 60% eidetically
but knew only 10% at the third-grade level and 0% at the fourth-grade
level. The 50% correct criterion is, therefore, at the second-grade level
(i.e., 60% meets the criterion of 50% or better).

The decoding mode in this case is relatively more phonetic: The patient was able to pick up many words in the P column after they were missed in the E column (P = phonetically known words decoded within 10 seconds). The phonetic performance is high compared with eidetic performance. Good phonetic decoding is indicated when close to half of the words missed in the E column can be decoded (picked up) phonetically. In this case, the patient picked up two of two words at the first-grade level, three of four at the second-grade level, four of nine at the third-grade level, and four of 10 at the fourth-grade level. Relatively good phonetic decoding is also indicated by the fact that the patient's eidetic decoding was only at the second-grade level, but he advanced to the fourth-grade level by phonetically decoding some words.

Encoding

Encoding is the portion of the DDT in which the patient is asked to spell words dictated by the clinician. In Case 1, the words selected by the clinician depend on the patient's basal, which is primer. This is found by the 10 odd-numbered E words going down from the second-grade level to lower levels. Words are also selected by finding the ceiling. In this case it is the fourth grade, 10 U words, odd or even, going up from the second-grade level to higher levels. These levels are clustered around the patient's eidetic decoding level. This patient's decoding level is at the second grade (50% correct criterion). From this level the dictation begins for E and U words.

Spelling to Basal (Eidetic Challenge)

For the eidetic encoding challenge, the clinician dictates words starting at the second grade (in this case) and moving to lower grade levels. The first word dictated is *rolled*. This word was selected because it was eidetically decoded by the patient (i.e., the patient recognized it and pronounced it in ≤2 seconds) and because it is odd numbered and thus phonetically irregular. The next word, *city*, meets the same criteria. These words, by the way, are considered phonetically irregular because they can be spelled in various ways (e.g., *rold* or *sity*). The next eight words that qualify for the eidetic encoding challenge are uncle, does, here, funny, guess, call, money, and came (Figure 10.2). (The word *came* is considered phonetically irregular for a first-grade student because the child may not have learned the phonetic rule of the marker *e* by that time.) These 10 words were chosen because they are eidetically pure, that is, the patient must have eidetic revisualization ability to spell the words correctly because he cannot rely on phonetics for help in spelling the words. The use of 10 words also establishes the basal level. To dictate fewer than 10 words would be insufficient for validity of evaluation of eidetic encoding. To give more than 10 words (beyond the basal) would also introduce the question of validity because the words become easier as the grade level lowers.

Grapheme — Nemkinesia Testing
(Writing Numbers and Letters by Examinee)

1 2 3 4 5 6 7 8 9 10

A B C D E F G H I J K L M N O P Q R S

T U V W X Y Z

a b c d e f g h i j k l m n o p q r s t u

v w x y z

Encoding (Spelling by Examinee)

Flash-Known Words — Non-phonetic (odd numbered) words only.		Unknown Words — Either phonetic (even-numbered) or non-phonetic (odd numbered) words.	
Rold	(rolled)	lisun	c
Sity	(city)	bisnis	c
Unkal	(uncle)	belev	c
dus	(does)	have	c
here	c	Shud	c
fune	(funny)	desh	(dish)
ges	(guess)	delit	c
cal	(call)	familyr	c
mone	(money)	Purpls	(pupils)
Came	c	sord	c
	20%		80%

FIGURE 10.2 Results of testing for dysnemkinesia and encoding in Case 1.

As mentioned earlier in this book, written expressive language (spelling in this case) is the most difficult of all forms of linguistic expression (more difficult than listening, speaking, and reading). Therefore words at and below the patient's eidetic decoding level are dictated for the eidetic encoding challenge. More difficult words are selected for the phonetic challenge.

Spelling to Ceiling (Phonetic Challenge)

The phonetic challenge presents unknown (U column) words for dictation (words that have not been decoded by the patient, either eidetically or phonetically and are, therefore, not in the patient's reading vocabulary). The phonetic encoding challenge is pure in that no eidetic strategy is presumed to help with the spelling of the dictated word. Increasingly difficult words are presented, starting at the patient's decoding level and progressing to higher grade levels to ensure that the patient truly does not know how to spell the words eidetically. The intent in the phonetic encoding challenge is to have the patient write a reasonably good phonetic equivalent of the dictated word. In this case, the first word dictated was *listen* (see Figure 10.2). The patient wrote it as *lisun*, which is phonetically acceptable. Other correct responses for the phonetic encoding challenge are *bisnis* (business), *belev* (believe), *heve* (heavy), *shud* (should), *delit* (delight), *familyr* (familiar), and *sord* (soared). The two incorrect phonetic equivalents are *desh* (dish) and *purels* (pupils). The decision to score *desh* as incorrect is a close call because there is not a tremendous difference between the sounds of the short *e* and the short *i*. The clinician in this case probably decided that this 11-year-old fifth grader should have been able to discern the difference. Regardless, the inter-rater reliability (between examiners using the DDT) is very high when judging acceptable phonetic equivalents. We have found it to be approximately 98%, even in newly trained clinicians.[2]

Interpretation of Results

The full instructions for administering the DDT are presented in the instruction manual and in the accompanying audiotape cassette. The ideas behind evaluation of results, however, are presented here to illustrate the principles of this direct method of testing and diagnosing dyslexia.

Grapheme-nemkinesia testing is shown in the upper portion of Figure 10.2. In this case, dysnemkinesia was ruled out because there were no reversals. One reason for having the patient undergo grapheme-nemkinesia testing first is to ensure that the necessary visual-motor skills are intact. Encoding testing would be invalid if the examinee could not write the numbers and letters, either because of poor visual-motor skills or lack of knowledge of these symbols. The patient also gains confidence and is less likely to feel threatened by the more challenging tasks of decoding and encoding testing. This is critical for a dyslexic patient who fears oral reading and writing tasks. Writing numbers is a relatively easy task, even for most dyslexic individuals, and helps the patient to warm up for further testing. Writing uppercase letters is a bit more challenging but usually not intimidating enough to threaten the patient. Writing lowercase letters is the most challenging of the three portions of the grapheme-nemkinesia testing; even here, most patients are sufficiently warmed up to the testing procedure by this time that anxiety is considerably reduced. Of the thousands of individuals we have tested, none has shown so much anxiety that testing had to be stopped. On one occasion, however, testing had to be suspended momentarily because a child's parents were in the testing room along with several other observers. Usually this does not present a problem, but it may be wise in some testing situations to be alone with the examinee.

In Figure 10.2, the eidetic encoding results are shown on the lower left. Correct responses are marked with a *c*, and incorrect responses are indicated by having the word correctly spelled in parentheses next to the misspelled one. In this case, the patient had two of 10 correct, or 20%. This is evaluated as moderate dyseidesia according to the criteria in the DDT instruction manual. The recording of this assessment is shown in Figure 10.3. (The encoding results are tied in with the decoding results to interpret severity of dyslexia.) Figure 10.2 (lower right) also shows the results of phonetic encoding, in which the patient had eight of 10 correct responses. The 80% score is normal.

Dysphonesia

Testing for dysphonetic dyslexia is the same as that described above for dyseidesia.

Decoding

An example of decoding is shown in the case of a 9-year-old in the fourth grade who is reading at the second-grade level in school (Case 2, Figure 10.4). From the discussion of decoding level in Case 1, it can be ascertained that the eidetic decoding level is at the second grade, with a basal eidetic decoding level at the primer level and the ceiling at mid–third grade. (Note that all grades above primer are considered midyear levels.) The decoding mode is relatively less phonetic (possibly more eidetic) because very few words were decoded phonetically; in fact, the patient picked up no words beyond first-grade level.

Encoding

The patient's eidetic and phonetic encoding responses (Figure 10.5) clearly reveal a dysphonetic pattern. She correctly wrote eight of 10 words on the eidetic encoding challenge but only 20% on the phonetic encoding challenge.

Interpretation of Results

According to the tables in the DDT instruction manual, the severity of the dysphonesia is moderate. Figure 10.6 shows the recording of these

INTERPRETATION RECORDING FORM

Dyslexia Determination Test (DDT)   Date _____

Examinee's
Name _____   Birth   AGE   Grade
                                          Date _____ Yrs. _11_ Mos. _4_   Placement _5Th_

History Summary: _Reading below grade level in school_

I. | **Grapheme-Nemkinesis Testing** | (Comments:) _Normal_

II. | **Results of Decoding:** | Form A ☑ Form B ☐

Highest grade level of sight-word recognition (50%) ___ 2nd

Number of Flash-Known words (at DDT grade level) ___ 6

Decoding Mode: Relatively more phonetic ☑   Relatively equal ☐

Relatively more eidetic ☐   Comments: _____

III. | **Results of Encoding**

Spelling of FLASH-KNOWN words for evaluation of DYSEIDESIA (using words that are DDT grade level and below for testing of ability of "re-visualization" of words). *Comments and results:* _____

___ 20% (moderate severity)

Spelling of UNKNOWN words (for phonetic equivalents) for evaluation of DYSPHONESIA (using words that are DDT grade level and above for testing of "phonetic word analysis," ability. *Comments and results:* _____

___ 80% (Normal)

DYSPHONEIDESIA (Dysphonesia and Dyseidesia). *Comments:* _____

Observation of behavior during writing (e.g., reversals, poor posture, poor pencil grip, slow speed of writing, poor eye-hand coordination, lack of fine motor control):

Interpretation (Synthesis of the results of the above testing)

0. ☐ No dyslexia (No dyslexic pattern found)
1. ☐ Dysnemkinesia
2. ☐ Dysphonesia
3. ☑ Dyseidesia _moderate_
4. ☐ Dysphoneidesia
5. ☐ Dysnemkinphonesia
6. ☐ Dysnemkineidesia
7. ☐ Dysnemkinphoneidesia

Comments: _Refer for educational assessment in school_

Signature of examiner: _____ Date _____

FIGURE 10.3 *Interpretation of results indicating moderately severe dyseidetic dyslexia in* Case 1.

---

results. Note that this patient reversed the number 7, which indicates a mild dysnemkinetic pattern. Also noteworthy is the substitution of the capital *D* for lowercase *d*, which indicates letter reversal problems. The combined diagnosis is therefore dysnemkinphonesia, with the dysnemkinetic component being mild and the dysphonetic component moderate. Although this dysphonetic component handicaps reading, writing, and spelling, the mild dysnemkinetic component is probably not a significant disability.

Date _____

DDT Decoding Patterns for FORM A
RECORDING PAGE

Examinee's Name _____

Birth Date _____ Yrs. _9_ Mos. _4_

AGE _____

Grade Placement _4Th_

Odd Numbered Words — Non Phonetic
Even Numbered Words — Phonetic

	p-primer	E	P	U		primer	E	P	U		1st	E	P	U		2nd	E	P	U
1	green				1	are				1	money				1	does			
2	an				2	yes				2	him				2	ask			
3	look				3	ready				3	call				3	listen			
4	go				4	did				4	if				4	just			
5	mother				5	lock				5	guess				5	uncle			
6	no				6	up				6	fast				6	sled			
7	said				7	black				7	funny				7	city			
8	stop				8	on				8	we				8	step			
9	ball				9	came				9	here				9	rolled			
10	in				10	it				10	with				10	wet			
	Totals					Totals	8	1	1		Totals	5	2	3		Totals	5	0	5

	3rd	E	P	U		4th	E	P	U		5th	E	P	U		6th	E	P	U
1	business				1	delight				1	height				1	badge			
2	lamp				2	human				2	invent				2	abandon			
3	believe				3	familiar				3	doubt				3	conceited			
4	jump				4	pupils				4	planted				4	melting			
5	heavy				5	soared				5	position				5	foreign			
6	path				6	trunk				6	grand				6	album			
7	laugh				7	rough				7	contagious				7	knapsack			
8	drink				8	whisk				8	handed				8	varnish			
9	should				9	glisten				9	vowed				9	decisions			
10	dish				10	prison				10	ambush				10	shifted			
	Totals	2	0	8		Totals					Totals					Totals			

	7—8	E	P	U		9—12	E	P	U		College	E	P	U
1	coolie				1	heinous				1	homologous			
2	edit				2	minus				2	emigrant			
3	graciously				3	graduation				3	homeopathy			
4	blunt				4	detested				4	subabdominal			
5	tomorrow				5	pollute				5	rheostat			
6	abhor				6	digit				6	admonish			
7	trudge				7	snuggle				7	demagogue			
8	devoted				8	prevalent				8	demented			
9	aeronautic				9	exonerate				9	euphony			
10	abolish				10	bonus				10	minuet			
	Totals					Totals					Totals			

Column Designations

"E" — Flash Known (Eidetic)
"P" — Untimed Known (Phonetic)
"U" — Unknown Words

Results of Decoding — FORM A

Highest grade level of sight word recognition (50% Flash Known) __2nd__

Number of Flash-Known words at DDT Grade Level __5__

Decoding Mode:

Relatively more phonetic ☐   Relatively more eidetic ☑   Relatively equal ☐

Comments: _____

_____

_____

Examiner: _____   Date: _____

FIGURE 10.4 *Decoding results in 9-year-old in fourth grade (Case 2).*

Dysphoneidesia

The mixed type of dyslexia characterized by both dyseidetic and dys-phonetic patterns is known as *dysphoneidesia*. Because two types are involved, this type of dyslexia is often more handicapping than a single type of either dyseidesia or dysphonesia. There are exceptions, of

Grapheme — Nemkinesia Testing
(Writing Numbers and Letters by Examinee)

1 2 3 4 5 6 Γ 8 9 10

A B C D E F G H i J K L M N O P Q R S t U
v w x y Z

a b c D e F g h i j k l m n o p Q r s t u v
w x y z

Encoding (Spelling by Examinee)

Flash-Known Words — Non-phonetic (odd numbered) words only.		Unknown Words — Either phonetic (even-numbered) or non-phonetic (odd numbered) words.	
City	c	Sak	(ask)
doES	c	listn	(listen)
hErE	c	unkl	c
Funny	c	Slab	(sled)
GnES	(guess)	rolled	c
tall	c	besas	(business)
Mone	(money)	LaP	(lamp)
Came	c	bede	(believe)
Lock	c	hadxe	(heavy)
are	c	laxuh	(laugh)
	80%		20%

FIGURE 10.5 *Results of testing for dysnemkinesia and encoding in Case 2.*

course, and a mild dysphoneidetic dyslexia may be less handicapping than either a marked dyseidesia or a marked dysphonesia. In general, dysphoneidesia is most handicapping, followed by dyseidesia, and then dysphonesia, with dysnemkinesia being the least handicapping of all types of dyslexia.

INTERPRETATION RECORDING FORM
Dyslexia Determination Test (DDT)

Date _____

Examinee's Name _____

Birth Date _____ Yrs. _9_ Mos. _4_   **AGE**   Grade Placement _4th_

History Summary: _Poor reader, often substitutes words when reading aloud._ _Transposes letters, e.g., solw for slow, and reverses letters and numbers._

I. | **Grapheme-Nemkinesis Testing** | (Comments:) _Several upper case substitutions when_ _when alphabet in lower case. One reversal, mild dysnemkinesia_

II. | **Results of Decoding:** | Form A ☑   Form B ☐

Highest grade level of sight-word recognition (50%) _2nd_

Number of Flash-Known words (at DDT grade level) _5_

Decoding Mode: Relatively more phonetic ☐ ,   Relatively equal ☐

Relatively more eidetic ☑   Comments: _____

III. | **Results of Encoding**

Spelling of FLASH-KNOWN words for evaluation of DYSEIDESIA (using words that are DDT grade level and below for testing of ability of "re-visualization" of words). *Comments and results:* _____

80% (normal)

Spelling of UNKNOWN words (for phonetic equivalents) for evaluation of DYSPHONESIA (using words that are DDT grade level and above for testing of "phonetic word analysis," ability. *Comments and results:* _____

20% (moderate)

DYSPHONEIDESIA (Dysphonesia and Dyseidesia). *Comments:* _____

Observation of behavior during writing (e.g., reversals, poor posture, poor pencil grip, slow speed of writing, poor eye-hand coordination, lack of fine motor control):

Interpretation (Synthesis of the results of the above testing)

0. ☐ No dyslexia (No dyslexic pattern found)
1. ☐ Dysnemkinesia
2. ☐ Dysphonesia
3. ☐ Dyseidesia
4. ☐ Dysphoneidesia
5. ☑ Dysnemkinphonesia _mild dysnemkinesia with moderate dysphonesia_
6. ☐ Dysnemkineidesia
7. ☐ Dysnemkinphoneidesia

Comments: _Refer to school for further assessment by resource_ _specialist and school psychologist._

Signature of examiner: _____ Date _____

FIGURE 10.6 *Interpretation of results indicating mild dysnemkinesia with moderate dysphonesia (i.e., dysnemkinphonesia) in Case 2.*

Figure 10.7 shows the decoding efforts of a 13-year-old in the seventh grade who is decoding at the third-grade level (Case 3). Both eidetic and phonetic decoding appear to be poor. Figure 10.8 shows the patient's poor eidetic and phonetic encoding. Results are recorded on the Interpretation Recording Form of the DDT (Figure 10.9).

Date _____

DDT Decoding Patterns for FORM A
RECORDING PAGE

Examinee's
Name _____

Birth
Date _____

AGE _____
Yrs. _13_ Mos. _3_

Grade
Placement _7 7h_

Odd Numbered Words — Non Phonetic
Even Numbered Words — Phonetic

	p-primer	E	P	U		primer	E	P	U		1st	E	P	U		2nd	E	P	U
1	green				1	are				1	money	●			1	does	●		
2	an				2	yes				2	him	●			2	ask	●		
3	look				3	ready				③	call	●			3	listen		●	
4	go				4	did				4	if				4	just	●		
5	mother				5	lock				5	guess		●		5	uncle			
6	no				6	up				6	fast			●	6	sled	●		
7	said				7	black				⑦	funny	●			⑦	city	●		
8	stop				8	on				8	we	●			8	step	●		
9	ball				9	came				⑨	here	●			⑨	rolled	●		
10	in				10	it				10	with			●	10	wet	●		
	Totals					Totals					Totals	7	2	1		Totals	8	2	0

	3rd	E	P	U		4th	E	P	U		5th	E	P	U		6th	E	P	U
①	business	●			1	delight			●	1	height				1	badge			
2	lamp	●			2	human			●	2	invent				2	abandon			
③	believe	●			3	familiar			●	3	doubt				3	conceited			
4	jump	●			4	pupils			●	4	planted				4	melting			
⑤	heavy	●			5	soared			●	5	position				5	foreign			
6	path	●			6	trunk			●	6	grand				6	album			
⑦	laugh	●			7	rough			●	7	contagious				7	knapsack			
8	should			●	8	whisk	●			8	handed				8	varnish			
9	should				9	glisten			●	9	vowed				9	decisions			
10	dish	●			10	prison			●	10	ambush				10	shifted			
	Totals	9	0	1		Totals	0	1	9		Totals					Totals			

	7—8	E	P	U		9—12	E	P	U		College	E	P	U
1	coolie				1	heinous				1	homologous			
2	edit				2	minus				2	emigrant			
3	graciously				3	graduation				3	homeopathy			
4	blunt				4	detested				4	subabdominal			
5	tomorrow				5	pollute				5	rheostat			
6	abhor				6	digit				6	admonish			
7	trudge				7	snuggle				7	demagogue			
8	devoted				8	prevalent				8	demented			
9	aeronautic				9	exonerate				9	euphony			
10	abolish				10	bonus				10	minuet			
	Totals					Totals					Totals			

Column Designations

"E" — Flash Known
(Eidetic)
"P" — Untimed Known
(Phonetic)
"U" — Unknown Words

Results of Decoding — FORM A

Highest grade level of sight word recognition (50% Flash Known) _3 rd_
Number of Flash-Known words at DDT Grade Level _9_

Decoding Mode:

Relatively more phonetic ☐   Relatively more eidetic ☐   Relatively equal ☑

Comments: _____
_____
_____
_____

Examiner: _____   Date: _____

FIGURE 10.7 *Decoding results of testing of a 13-year-old in seventh grade (Case 3).*

Other Types of Dyslexia

Evaluation of reversals is discussed previously in this chapter and also
in Chapter 9, Directionality for Numbers and Letters, in regard to the

Grapheme — Nemkinesia Testing
(Writing Numbers and Letters by Examinee)

1 2 3 4 5 6 7 8 9 10

A B C D E F G H I J K L M N O P Q R S
T U V W X Y Z

a b c d e f g h i j k l m n o p q r
s t u v w x y z

Encoding (Spelling by Examinee)

Flash-Known Words — Non-phonetic (odd numbered) words only.		Unknown Words — Either phonetic (even-numbered) or non-phonetic (odd numbered) words.	
Laf	(laugh)	Suold	(should)
have	(heavy)	Delit	(c
BeLive	(believe)	heum	(human)
Bussing	(business)	fmeler	(familiar)
Rolled	c	Pol	(pupils)
cily	(city)	Sor	(soared)
Duss	(does)	Track	(trunk)
here	c	ref	(rough)
funing	(funny)	Glish	e
Called	(call)	Peris	(prison)
	20%		20%

FIGURE 10.8 *Results of testing for dysnemkinesia and encoding in Case 3.*

Gardner Reversals Frequency Test.[11] The Gardner test for reversals is a good adjunct to the DDT's grapheme-nemkinesia testing for dysnemkinesia. The dysnemkinetic type is colloquially called *motoric dyslexia*. It is infrequently found in isolation but is most often a component of a mixed type. Because there are three basic types of dyslexia (dyseidesia

INTERPRETATION RECORDING FORM
Dyslexia Determination Test (DDT)

Date _____

Examinee's
Name _____

Birth
Date _____ Yrs. _13_ $\frac{AGE}{Mos.}$ _3_

Grade
Placement _7Th_

History Summary: _Reading much below grade level_____

I. | Grapheme-Nemkinesis Testing | (Comments:) _No reversals but several_

lower and upper case confusions. No indication of dysnemkinesia.

II. | Results of Decoding: | Form A ☑   Form B ☐

Highest grade level of sight-word recognition (50%) ___3_____

Number of Flash-Known words (at DDT grade level) ___9_____

Decoding Mode: Relatively more phonetic ☐   Relatively equal ☑

Relatively more eidetic ☐   Comments: _____

III. | Results of Encoding |

Spelling of FLASH-KNOWN words for evaluation of DYSEIDESIA (using words that are DDT grade level and below for testing of ability of "re-visualization" of words). *Comments and results:* _____

20% (moderate severity)

Spelling of UNKNOWN words (for phonetic equivalents) for evaluation of DYSPHONESIA (using words that are DDT grade level and above for testing of "phonetic word analysis," ability. *Comments and results:* _____

20% (moderate severity)

DYSPHONEIDESIA (Dysphonesia and Dyseidesia). *Comments:* _____

Mixed Type, moderately severe in each

Observation of behavior during writing (e.g., reversals, poor posture, poor pencil grip, slow speed of writing, poor eye-hand coordination, lack of fine motor control):

Interpretation (Synthesis of the results of the above testing)

0. ☐ No dyslexia (No dyslexic pattern found)
1. ☐ Dysnemkinesia
2. ☐ Dysphonesia
3. ☐ Dyseidesia
4. ☑ Dysphoneidesia _moderate_
5. ☐ Dysnemkinphonesia
6. ☐ Dysnemkineidesia
7. ☐ Dysnemkinphoneidesia

Comments: _Referral for educational testing and counseling._

Signature of examiner: _____   Date _____

FIGURE 10.9 *Interpretation of results indicating moderately severe dysphoneidesia in Case 3.*

or visual type, dysphonesia or auditory type, and dysnemkinesia or motoric type), there are seven possible permutations. The four mixed types are dysphoneidesia, dysnemkinphonesia, dysnemkineidesia, and dysnemkinphoneidesia. Because these long Greek-rooted names are difficult for many patients to say and comprehend, the clinician may resort to the more practical, but imprecise and not completely accurate, terms of visual, auditory, and motoric dyslexia. It is easier to explain to a patient or parent that the dyslexia, for example, is motoric and auditory than to refer to the diagnosis as dysnemkinphonesia.

Prevalence of dyslexia is discussed in Chapter 3. As a general rule, about one-third of all dyslexics have dyseidesia, about one-third have dysphonesia, and approximately one-third have combined types.

Other Tests for Dyslexia

Materials for testing[1, 2, 4–10] and therapy[3] compatible with the DDT are listed in Table 10.1. The name of the test or screener is given with the appropriate age or grade level for testing. Full instructions and background information are provided in the instruction manuals for each test (see Chapters 1–3 and other sources[12–24]).

Summary

The DDT is widely used for testing dyslexia. The first part of the test involves checking for written reversals of numbers and letters. The second part tests the mode of decoding words: eidetic or phonetic. The third part of the test assesses whether encoding is eidetic or phonetic. Direct diagnostic testing is necessary to determine both the type and severity of dyslexia. Case examples of several of the seven types of dyslexia are presented. Various tests similar to the DDT, which are appropriate for various ages and languages, are listed.

References

1. Boder E, Jarrico S. The Boder Test of Reading and Spelling Patterns. New York: Grune & Stratton, 1982.
2. Griffin JR, Walton HN. Dyslexia Determination Test (DDT) (2nd ed rev). Los Angeles: Instructional Materials and Equipment Distributors, 1987.
3. Griffin JR, Walton HN. Therapy in Dyslexia and Reading Problems. Los Angeles: Instructional Materials and Equipment Distributors, 1985.
4. Griffin JR, Walton HN, Lind YG. Spanish Screening Version of the Dyslexia Determination Test (DDT). Los Angeles, CA: Instructional Materials and Equipment Distributors, 1989.
5. Griffin JR, Walton HN, Ward L. French Screening Version of the DDT. Los Angeles: Reading and Perception Therapy Center, 1995.
6. Griffin JR, Walton HN, Christenson GN. The Dyslexia Screener (TDS). Culver City, CA: Reading and Perception Therapy Center, 1988.
7. Griffin JR, Christenson GN, Walton HN. Adult Dyslexia Test (ADT). Los Angeles: Reading and Perception Therapy Center, 1990.

8. Griffin JR, Walton HN. Dyslexia Screener for First-Graders (DSF). Culver City, CA: Reading and Perception Therapy Center, 1990.

9. Wesson MD, Griffin JR, Christenson GN. Predyslexia Letter Coding Test (PLCT). Culver City, CA: Reading and Perception Therapy, 1994.

10. Christenson GN, Erickson GB, Griffin JR, et al. Home Dyslexia Screening Test (HDST). Hudson, WI: Christenson Therapy Center, 1996.

11. Gardner RA. Gardner Reversals Frequency Test. Cresskill, NJ: Creative Therapeutics, 1979.

12. Christenson GN, Griffin JR, Wesson MD. Optometry's role in reading disabilities: resolving the controversy. J Am Optom Assoc 1990;61:363–71.

13. Johnson DJ, Myklebust HR. Learning Disabilities. New York: Grune & Stratton, 1967;173.

14. Boder E. Developmental dyslexia: a diagnostic approach based on three atypical reading patterns. Dev Med Child Neurol 1973;15:663–87.

15. Camp BW, Dolcourt JL. Reading and spelling in good and poor readers. J Learn Disabil 1977;10:300–7.

16. Geschwind N. Specializations of the human brain. Sci Am 1979;241:180–99.

17. Duffy FH, Denkle MB, Bartels PH, et al. Dyslexia: automated diagnosis by computerized classifications of brain electrical activity. Ann Neurol 1980;7:421–8.

18. Shallice T. Phonological agraphia and the lexical route in writing. Brain (Oxford) 1981;104:413–29.

19. Roeltgen DP, Sevush S, Heilman KM. Phonological agraphia: writing by the lexical-semantic route. Neurology 1983;33:755–65.

20. Hynd GW, Hynd CR. Dyslexia: neuroanatomical/neurolinguistic perspectives. Reading Res Q 1984;19:482–98.

21. Roeltgen DP, Heilman KM. Lexical agraphia—further support for the two-system hypothesis of linguistic agraphia. Brain (Oxford) 1984;107:811–27.

22. Temple CM. New approaches to the developmental dyslexias. Adv Neurol 1984;42:223–32.

23. Flynn JM, Deering WM. Subtypes of dyslexia: investigation of Boder's classification system using quantitative neurophysiology. Dev Med Child Neurol 1989;31:215–23.

24. Semrund-Clikeman M. Neuropsychological Evidence for Subtypes in Developmental Dyslexia. In LR Putnam (ed), How to Become a Better Reading Teacher. Englewood Cliffs, NJ: Merrill, 1996;43–52.

IV. Therapy for Reading Dysfunction

11   Optometric Treatment

Specific approaches to therapy are based on testing results. The optometrist's therapeutic regimen for reading dysfunction (RD) consists of *vision therapy*, to improve visual skills efficiency (VSE) and to remedy visual-perceptual-motor (VPM) problems, and *educational therapy* for reading problems from other causes, such as dyslexia. The focus of this chapter is the use of vision therapy to remedy vision deficiencies that can cause general (nonspecific) reading problems and contribute to specific reading problems (dyslexia). Educational therapy is discussed in Chapter 12.

Vision Therapy Principles

Vision therapy is a process of using binocular and VPM experiences that serve as developmentally appropriate tasks for the patient to accomplish. The therapist encourages, guides, and challenges the patient during functional training procedures. The therapist does not cure the patient as much as the patient cures himself or herself through awareness of the internal strategies necessary to accomplish the visual task (i.e., the vision training technique). Through practice and intersensory integration (e.g., auditory-visual integration), the task becomes automatic and VPM maturity may be achieved. Effective therapy cannot be performed strictly on a home-training basis. Active therapy with a trained therapist is absolutely necessary to guide the patient to the level of self-awareness of processing and eventually to automaticity of processing.

Vision therapy can be divided into treatment for *VSE* (accommodation, binocularity, and eye movement function), and *VPM* therapy. Both areas are covered in this text, and other texts have been written on these topics.[1–4]

Rationale for Effective Vision Therapy

Before our discussion of therapeutic objectives, techniques, and sequencing, it is necessary to establish the rationale for administering vision therapy. The mechanisms for treating vision-related reading problems are presented from three perspectives:

1. Documented support for the efficacy of vision therapy.
2. Use of auditory-visual integrative therapy as a complement to standard vision therapy and to facilitate development of selective attention abilities.
3. The possible effect of vision therapy on magnocellular processing (M-pathway) deficits (see Chapter 4, Information Output from the Retina, for a discussion of M-pathway deficits and Chapter 5, Tinted or Attenuating Filters).

In 1986, a task force composed of experts in the field published an extensive report on research that indicated high effectiveness of therapy to improve visual functions.[5] Vision therapy is designed as a supplement to, rather than a substitute for, classroom activities. Good VSE and VPM skills for information processing are essential for reading improvement.

Auditory-visual integration correlates with reading achievement in the early grades.[6] Many vision therapy techniques in this text incorporate the use of a metronome. This combination, for example, making a saccadic eye movement with each click of the metronome, helps the patient match visual and auditory stimuli, thus facilitating integration between the two sense modalities. Auditory-visual techniques also foster the use of appropriate attentive mechanisms, such as proper arousal levels, filtering of stimuli for processing, and initiation of appropriate task responses. This integrative ability has a direct bearing on the development of the basic visual processing skills important for reading achievement.

The relation between visual processing therapy and attention is germane to attention-deficit disorder (ADD) and attention-deficit hyperactivity disorder (ADHD). We believe that controversy about accurate diagnosis of ADD and ADHD along with the desire to "do something" for the child who has trouble paying attention in school can lead to the overuse of psychostimulant medications. It is likely that some children diagnosed as ADD or ADHD may actually suffer from vision problems that impair the ability to attend, such as accommodative insufficiency, directionality problems, and poor auditory-visual integration. Multidisciplinary teamwork is critical for successful management of a child with RD, especially when ADD or ADHD is a factor.

Research evidence indicates that a magnocellular (transient system) processing deficit is highly prevalent among children with severe reading problems.[7-10] Although there is no evidence relating this deficit to dyseidetic dyslexia, Borsting et al.[11] did find a possible relation between dysphoneidesia and a magnocellular deficit, namely, that the dysphonetic component could be the relative factor. The presence of this deficit may also be significant as an indicator of vision problems that contribute to general reading problems.

The possibility of a magnocellular deficit in dysphoneidesia is logical, considering the investigations of Galaburda,[12] who showed that the brains of individuals with severe dyslexia have abnormal neural development in the left hemisphere. Galaburda found large numbers of ectopias (small loci of disorganized groups of neurons) and dysplasias (focally distorted cortical architecture) primarily in the area of the left temporoparietal lobe. Galaburda's criteria for including the brains of subjects in his study are congruous with the characteristics of marked dysphoneidesia. Manifestation of dysphoneidesia may be due to ectopias and dysplasias in the dominant temporoparietal lobe; these abnormalities may cause the characteristic reading and spelling deficiencies and appear to be related to the magnocellular processing deficit often noted in the literature.[7-13] Anatomically this is logical because the magnocellular pathway extends through the middle temporal area to the posterior parietal cortex.[10] Further research is needed for clarification.

Does vision therapy have a beneficial effect on the imbalance in parallel processing caused by the magnocellular deficit? Indirect evidence indicates that it could. Filters that attenuate contrast seem to reestablish the balance between the M- and P-pathways, supposedly eliminating visual persistence and the accompanying symptoms of blurred print, "swimming" letters, and unstable images.[10] Scheiman et al.[14] investigated a population of "positive filter responders" and found that 95% had accommodative and binocular problems, such as accommodative insufficiency and convergence insufficiency. It is conceivable that VSE problems are related to a parallel processing deficit. Tentative support for this concept is provided by Garzia and Sesma.[10] Cardinal et al.[15] reviewed the literature on the Irlen treatment with tinted lenses and concluded that its scientific basis is questionable, and that tinted lenses or overlays did not result in better and faster reading. We recommend vision therapy rather than the use of tinted lenses for RD patients with VSE problems. (Refer to Case 5 in Chapter 12.)

Multidisciplinary Approach

We present a concept of multidisciplinary care that incorporates a neurologic model, the roles of professionals on the therapeutic management team, and a therapeutic synthesis.

Mesulam[16] described a "cortical network for directed attention" that can be reconciled with our model of cognitive-linguistic processing (eidetic and phonetic coding). Mesulam demonstrated that the posterior parietal lobe receives and organizes input from four sites in the brain: (1) the retinogeniculocortical pathway (visual input from the eyes to the visual cortex), (2) the reticular activating system (RAS) (arousal and attention input), (3) the parahippocampal gyrus of the limbic system (motivational relevance), and (4) the frontal lobe (motor planning). Figure 11.1 illustrates the areas involved in this system, which modulates the ability to direct attention to visual stimuli in the surrounding visual field. A description of the input to the posterior parietal lobe enables a more complete understanding of the nature of this system. In the retinogeniculocortical pathway, visual impulses received by the retina are processed and transmitted to the visual cortex. From here, impulses travel to the posterior parietal lobe to be processed with input from the other three brain areas involved. The aggregate of all four inputs provides the parietal lobe with a wealth of information that must be analyzed to select the most appropriate, motivationally relevant information. Based on these selected impulses, the individual responds with attentionally directed behavior (e.g., an appropriate saccade, a motor movement, increased peripheral awareness, or verbal responses). The RAS provides the appropriate level of attention, which varies according to RAS input from asleep to awake to alert to attentive.

The role of the parahippocampal gyrus (part of the limbic system) is to provide information on the motivational relevance of visual stimuli. To a person crossing a street, for example, a peripheral stimulus, such as a stationary object on the horizon, would likely be much less relevant than a car speeding toward the person (in the peripheral field).

Frontal lobe processing is involved in motor planning. For example, a man walking across the street while looking up at a building is peripherally aware of the curb as he approaches it, and plans to step over the curb without changing fixation from the upward gaze.

The frontal lobe, parahippocampal gyrus, and RAS all receive visual input as a stimulus for the attentional information they transmit to the posterior parietal lobe. The frontal lobe communicates independently with the limbic system. Thus, a complex integrated system of cortical

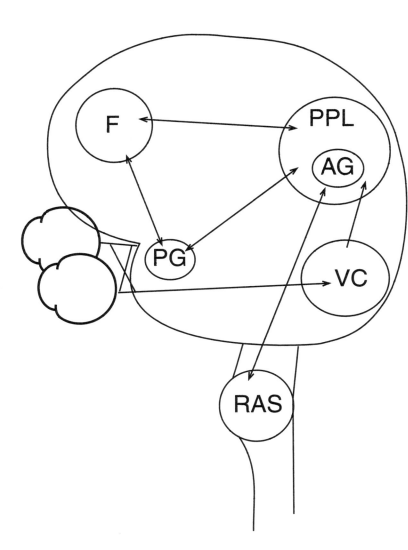

FIGURE 11.1
Schematic of the cortical system of directed visual attention. (F = frontal lobe; PG = parahippocampal gyrus; RAS = reticular activating system; VC = visual cortex; PPL = posterior parietal lobe; AG = angular gyrus.)

networking provides the information necessary for guiding visual behavior. Our highly simplified presentation provides context for the various therapies for reading problems.

The four areas of input into the posterior parietal lobe relate to at least four of the respective multidisciplinary professions involved in the care of individuals with RD: the retinogeniculocortical pathway relates to optometry, the RAS to medicine, the limbic system to psychology, and the frontal lobes to occupational therapy. The posterior parietal lobe function can be related to the teaching of decoding and encoding of words by education professionals.

Optometry is directly involved when vision problems require lens prescription or vision therapy. Medical treatment is frequently used in cases of poor attentional skills. Although we believe that stimulant medication for ADD and ADHD is often overprescribed, many properly selected patients do benefit from pharmacologic treatment. Psychologists are involved in treatment both as directors of psychoeducational assessment and counseling in the school system and as referral sources for primary emotional problems. Occupational therapists are often employed in school districts and as private practitioners to provide therapy to improve sensorimotor integration. Special educators are called on when it has been determined that traditional teaching methods are ineffective. We advocate careful consideration of referral to all appropriate team members when indicated by case history and clinical findings. Good multidisciplinary teamwork is critical to successful management of children with learning problems, particularly in cases of RD.

The cortical system of directed attention affects language skills for reading and writing (decoding and encoding). Visual impulses travel in an integrated cortical network through the parietal lobe for the purpose of directing attention. The area apparently responsible for providing sight-sound recognition in the coding of the written language lies in the angular gyrus of the posterior parietal lobe. Note that the neurologic substrates corresponding to functions treated by the various multidisciplinary team members all converge on the area (posterior parietal lobe) that simultaneously serves written language coding and directed attention. This is the area involved in dyseidesia, and in dysphonesia to some extent. Our model of neurobehaviorial function lends support to the clinical evidence demonstrating that patients with dyseidesia or dysphonesia require a structured, sequential multisensory (visual-auditory-kinesthetic) approach in educational therapy (see Chapter 12, under Specific Reading Dysfunction).

When dyslexia is ruled out and a nonspecific reading problem is apparent, optometric vision therapy or treatment by other multidisciplinary team members may be the principal treatment needed. The nature of therapy for dyslexia requires integration of visual perception, motor planning, kinesthetic processing, auditory processing, and the appropriate level of attention. Vision therapy uses these elements in concert to allow the child to develop age-appropriate VPM skills. It also serves as the foundation for multisensory language therapy when needed in the treatment of dyslexia.

An example of the above-mentioned "foundation" is offered in the case of a patient whose system of directed attention and written language processing has been compromised, such as a person with a stroke affecting the left cerebral cortex. In the individual with severely impaired language function, word comprehension may be increased when his or her fingers trace the letters. When touch, sight, and hearing are used simultaneously, language skills (both oral and written) may be reacquired. Although stroke patients and individuals with dyslexia are very different, both have an inefficiency of the neurophysiologic cortical network for directed attention that relates to language function. The multisensory combination of sight, sound, and touch allows sufficient input into the cortical network to serve as a "sensory trigger" to expedite language learning in stroke patients and in individuals with dyslexia.[17] Practically, this is achieved through VPM therapy in combination with structured, sequential, multisensory language therapy.

Vision Therapy Techniques

We divide vision therapy for RD into two broad categories: VSE and VPM therapy. See Chapter 9 for testing and assessment criteria. Equipment and sources can be found in the Appendix.

Sequence of Therapy

For the sake of brevity, specific procedures are presented in general performance terms. We present only a sample of the many procedures applicable to vision therapy for RD. Other texts can be consulted for more detailed information and additional vision training procedures.[1–4, 18] For a historic perspective, see Birnbaum's[19] review of the contributions of many pioneers in therapy techniques.

Therapy generally begins with training of VSE problems in the following order: (1) eye movements, (2) accommodation, and (3) vergence. A noteworthy exception to this rule occurs in patients with significant motor-planning or sensory-integrative problems. These patients are unable to handle the fine motor planning and integrative demands of the accommodative, vergence, and saccadic techniques. In the case of severe deficiency in these areas, referral for sensory-integrative occupational therapy may be indicated.[20] In the event of a motor or integrative problem, the therapist generally begins treatment sequencing with bilateral procedures, such as jumping jacks and windshield wipers, to facilitate motor planning. These gross motor movements are conducted in concert with the auditory beat of a metronome. After proficiency is developed, the patient, usually a child, may be ready to meet the demands of higher-level tasks involved in VSE procedures.

Concepts for the Therapist

The therapist may be the optometrist, a trained office assistant, or a helper (e.g., parent) at home. The therapist should be aware that simply having the patient perform a training technique does not constitute vision therapy. The optometrist must be directive and prescribe the appropriate treatment regimen. His or her assistant, ideally a certified optometric vision therapist, can then carry out much of the actual training techniques and instruct patients and parents on home training techniques. For the visual skill to be transformed into an efficient automatic process, the therapist must make the patient aware of the strategy necessary to accomplish the procedure. The training techniques introduce developmentally appropriate problems that the patient must solve. This requires the therapist to emphasize awareness of process. When administering a technique such as accommodative near-far rock, for example, the therapist engages the patient in a way that allows the patient to communicate the feeling involved in focusing on a very near target as opposed to a distant target. The near target may produce a feeling of "straining" or "zooming in." The art of vision therapy is teaching patients to master this awareness without telling the patient what it should feel like. The therapist must also serve as the motivator and source of positive feedback. Most patients with learning problems have experienced a great deal of frustration and failure. The therapist should therefore pursue the following sequence of reinforcement over the course of several therapy sessions: (1) initially praise the patient frequently for remotely appropriate visual performance; (2) as improvement is made, point out the patient's errors within the framework of the task and attempt not to discourage the patient's success, continue frequent praise; (3) with further increased proficiency, encourage the patient to catch his or her errors; and (4) encourage the patient to catch his or her errors and continue the training procedure without stopping. (Errors include getting "off beat" and not performing the task appropriately.)

Visual Skills Efficiency Training Techniques

VSE training techniques include those for saccadic eye movements, accommodation, and vergences. Deficiencies in these functions can cause or contribute to RD. We usually recommend that these functions be treated before training for any significant VPM deficiencies.

Saccadic Eye Movements

Saccadic therapy generally begins with gross saccadic activities and progresses to fine saccadic demands. These procedures can be done monocularly and binocularly. It is often advisable to improve monocular skills before binocular skills, but this may not be necessary if the monocular abilities are at an adequate level. During the early stages of training, accuracy is emphasized. Elimination of head movements is encouraged. Speed is encouraged after accuracy is optimal. During training, the use of a metronome helps to develop control and automaticity of saccades. For example, the patient performs a saccadic procedure in rhythm with a metronome set at 60 beats per minute so that the eyes fixate a new target each second.

Steps in Saccadic Therapy

1. Develop the patient's awareness of accurate and stable fixation (feedback may include afterimages on the fovea and verbal coaching by the therapist).

```
H T S R U Y O B N E

R A L V P S L E G Z

U R M C B S E R K T

E F H K D L M Z W A

W R K T G S X G U O

T R W J K G N C X S

R P K H F S X N V B

T C H F S A W M B R

L J G D E T X B C Z

M K H G E X Z W E X
```

FIGURE 11.2 *A custom-made Hart chart.*

2. Develop gross to fine saccades.
3. Develop accurate sequential (left-to-right) saccades.

Corner Saccades

The patient stands facing the center of a wall approximately 3 m away. The patient is instructed to fixate the four corners of the wall in the following order: upper-left, upper-right, lower-left, and lower-right corner. These gross saccades require the same directional movements as does reading English text. The therapist observes the patient's eyes and provides verbal feedback on accuracy of the saccades (undershooting, overshooting, or on target). Entoptic stimuli may increase feedback sensitivity; for example, an afterimage of a vertical line can be generated for the patient to monitor accuracy of foveal fixation.

Hart Chart Saccades

A special chart for training, devised by Dr. Walter Hart, is composed of an array of equally spaced random letters (Figure 11.2). The size of the letters and spacing between them can be altered to increase or decrease the difficulty of the saccadic task. An internal-row saccade procedure can be performed as follows: The patient is instructed to face the chart, which has been placed on a wall approximately 1 m from the patient, and call out the first and last letter in the top row. When the patient can do this with good speed and accuracy, he or she is told to call out the second letter and second-to-last letter in the row. This is repeated for the third letter, and so forth, until the patient is calling out the letters of the two middle columns of the chart. The next rows are fixated in the same manner. The demand progresses from gross to fine saccades. Many other variations of saccadic patterns can be used with Hart charts, such as reading every other letter in sequential rows.

Accommodation

Before binocular training is begun, monocular accommodative skills should be adequate. During the early stages of training, clarity is emphasized. Speed is encouraged only when clarity is consistently achieved. A metronome is added to the training tasks to help develop control and automaticity of accommodative responses. The patient must coordinate the focusing of each new target with the beat of the metronome.

Steps in Accommodative Therapy

1. Develop the patient's awareness of focusing effort.
2. Develop normal accommodative accuracy (stable, clear vision at various distances).
3. Develop normal accommodative amplitudes (generally at least 10.00 D for elementary school–aged children).
4. Develop normal accommodative facility monocularly (±2.00 D lens flipper) at a minimum of 10 cycles per minute (cpm) and then binocularly (±2.00 D lens flipper) with suppression check at a minimum of 5 cpm.

Near-Far Rock

Monocular accommodative facility training can be accomplished by having the patient look from far to near and from near to far, "rocking" between the two repeatedly. Many targets are suitable for this purpose, but the Hart chart is an excellent choice. A chart with large letters is attached to a wall about 3 m away from the patient, who holds a similar but much smaller chart with letters of reduced size. The patient occludes one eye and holds this smaller chart at his nearpoint of accommodation (e.g., 8 cm). When a letter on the chart can be seen clearly, the patient is instructed to look away to the far chart and attempt to clear a letter on it. Emphasis is placed on having the patient feel the difference between the focusing effort required at near versus far, that is, straining versus relaxing focus. When that is done successfully, the patient attempts to clear another letter on the smaller chart.

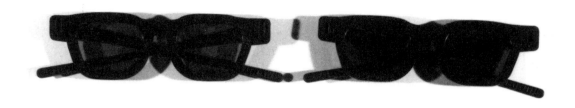

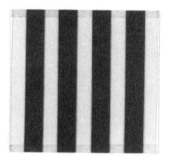 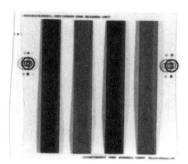

FIGURE 11.3   *Bar reading strips for monitoring suppression. The set on the left is vectographic; the set on the right is anaglyphic.*

Various patterns of letter sequencing (see Hart Chart Saccades above) can be prescribed for the patient to perform in the office and at home.

When monocular accommodative facility is fast and accurate (e.g., 10 cpm), the patient can begin binocular accommodative rock training. This is done in the same manner except that the nearpoint of binocular accommodation may be slightly more remote (e.g., 12 cm). The therapist monitors for suppression during binocular accommodative therapy, especially when a fundamental binocular anomaly exists, such as convergence insufficiency. In that case, vergence therapy may be needed before training for binocular accommodative rock facility.

Lens Flipper Rock

Accommodative rock can also be done using plus and minus lenses. The stimulatory phase occurs when the patient accommodates through a lens of minus power; the inhibitory phase is with a lens of plus power. Relatively low powers may be necessary in the beginning, but increased powers may be introduced gradually as accommodative facility improves with training. As in near-far rock, monocular training usually precedes binocular rock. The target should be small but suprathreshold, such as newsprint. For suppression monitoring with binocular rock, vectographic or anaglyphic bar reading strips are ideal (Figure 11.3).[1]

Vergences

Vergence training activities begin with gross convergence and continue with increasing demands on relative (fusional) vergence. As vergence ranges improve, activities that require rapid changes in relative vergence are emphasized. The goal is to ensure good vergence facility and stamina in the open environment.

Steps in Vergence Therapy

1. Develop gross convergence awareness (the feeling of straining for near binocular viewing versus relative relaxing for distant binocular viewing).
2. Develop physiologic diplopia (as in Brock string training, in which the beads that are not fixated appear double).
3. Develop voluntary convergence (ability to cross eyes without a near fixation target).
4. Eliminate suppression.
5. Develop normal sliding (gradually increasing target disparity) vergence ranges.
6. Develop fast and accurate vergence recoveries.

Pencil Push-ups

An ordinary pencil, pen, pointer stick, or fingertip can be used for target-advancement training. This procedure is useful for directly increasing gross (absolute) *convergence* and indirectly increasing fusional (relative) *convergence* abilities in cases of convergence insufficiency as well as for indirectly increasing fusional (relative) *divergence* abilities in cases of convergence excess.[1]

The patient is instructed to hold the fixation target at arm's length in the primary position of gaze and attempt to keep it clear. A small letter printed on the pencil is an excellent accommodative stimulus to monitor blur. The patient slowly moves the pencil toward his or her nose and reports when the letter on the pencil appears to blur and when it appears double. At this point, the patient should use mental effort to try to cross his or her eyes to see the letter on the pencil as single again. It may be necessary to move the pencil slowly away to regain fusion with clearness. Advancement of the target can then be resumed. This procedure is repeated several times. The goal is to keep the target clear and single at progressively closer distances.

Brock String Training

The Brock string[1] is a white cord strung with three different-colored beads. Brock string training is useful for increasing gross (absolute) convergence, monitoring suppression during vergence demands, increasing fusional convergence abilities in exophoric patients, and increasing fusional divergence abilities in cases of esophoria. The

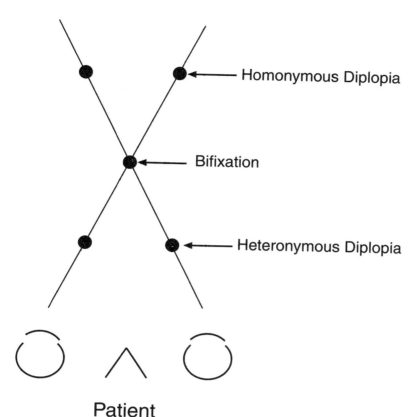

Homonymous Diplopia

Bifixation

Heteronymous Diplopia

Patient

FIGURE 11.4
Normal physiologic diplopia demon-strated with the Brock string.

patient is asked to hold one end of the string against the tip of his or her nose while the other end of the string is secured to a fixed object 2–3 m away. Initially, the beads are placed at approximately 20 cm, 50 cm, and 80 cm from the patient's nose.

The patient is asked to look at the middle bead and report how many strings are seen in front of the bead and how many strings are seen beyond the middle bead. If there is no suppression, two strings should be seen in front of the bead and two behind, forming an X pattern (Figure 11.4). This is normal physiologic diplopia. If this percept is reported, the patient is asked to say exactly where the strings appear to cross when looking at the middle bead. If the strings do not cross exactly at the bead, inaccurate bifixation is indicated. Very small vergence inac-curacies (fixation disparities) may be seen, such as the intersection of string images slightly in front of the fixated bead in the case of an esode-viation inaccuracy and slightly behind in an exodeviation inaccuracy.

The therapy goal is for the patient to fuse each bead easily, without any suppression or fixation disparity. Suppression is indicated by the disappearance of part or all of one string image. Distance and spacing of the beads can be adjusted to vary the vergence demands appropriately for each patient. A variety of other procedures can be performed with the Brock string, such as having the patient wear red-green filters and base-in or base-out prisms during training.

Vectographic and Tranaglyphic Targets

Numerous Vectograms and Tranaglyphs (anaglyphic targets) are commercially available (see Appendix). They come in two forms, either split for varying base-in and base-out demands for sliding vergences or fixed and invariable as to sliding vergence, sometimes with small step vergence demands. Vectographic targets are viewed with crossed-polarizing filters, and anaglyphic targets are viewed with red-green filters. A Dual Polachrome Illuminated Trainer (Bernell Corporation, South Bend, IN) is an effective device used for viewing vectographic targets during training. These procedures can improve second-degree (flat) and third-degree (stereopsis) sensory fusion while building motor fusion skills.

The patient wears the mutually excluding filters (e.g., crossed-polarizing filters) while viewing the target at 40 cm. Most targets have laterally separated portions to produce stereopsis from the effect of either crossed or uncrossed disparity. Split targets can be separated to increase the relative vergence demand smoothly for sliding vergence training. Two such pairs of Vectograms can be set up to allow training of step vergence skills to be trained, such as changing fixation from the top pair with base-in demand (to stimulate fusional divergence) to the bottom pair with base-out demand (to stimulate fusional convergence) (Figure 11.5). In the Vectograms and Tranaglyphs are targets used to monitor for suppression. The patient can be questioned about small-in large-out (SILO) effects as well. Perception of this size constancy phenomenon ensures that fusion is present, as in chiastopic fusion training.[1] The goal for the patient is to improve blur, break, and recovery responses to fusional convergence and divergence demands.

Aperture-Rule Trainer

The Aperture-Rule Trainer (ART) (Bernell Corporation, South Bend, IN) consists of a ruler base, a single- or double-window aperture, and a spiral-bound set of picture cards.[1] The single-window aperture is used for training fusional convergence; the double-window aperture is used for training fusional divergence. The ART requires some minor assembly, and instructions for ruler placement of the single or double aperture are on the picture cards.

The ART should be adjusted so that the appropriate end of the ruler touches the patient's nose. The first two cards in the set are used to assess suppression with the double aperture. Cards numbered 1–12 are separated to have increasing amounts of disparity. The prism diopter amount is determined by multiplying the card number by 2.5. For example, card 4 has 10^Δ of disparity. Controls within each picture card are used to monitor for suppression.

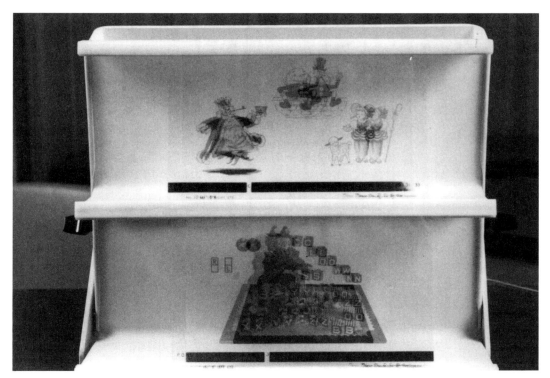

FIGURE 11.5   *Two variable Vectograms for use in step vergence training.*

The goal is for the patient to achieve fusion and clarity on progressively higher-numbered cards, up to card 12 with the single-window aperture and card 7 with the double aperture. Additionally, step vergence activities and activities with base-in prism with minus lenses and base-out prism with plus lenses can be performed with this instrument by using lens and prism flippers.

Chiastopic and Orthoptic Fusion

The Keystone Colored Circles or Eccentric Circles are fixed and variable targets, respectively, that can be used to train chiastopic and orthoptic fusion. These procedures develop sensory and motor fusion skills in the open environment. They are useful in improving fusional convergence with chiastopic activities and fusional divergence with orthoptic activities. Opaque stock cards are generally used for training chiastopic fusion (Figure 11.6) and clear acetate cards (Figure 11.7) are used for training orthoptic fusion.

The patient is instructed to hold the card or cards approximately 40 cm away from his or her face and to attempt to converge the eyes (look closer than the card) to achieve chiastopic fusion; to achieve orthoptic fusion, the patient is to diverge his or her eyes (look through the card).

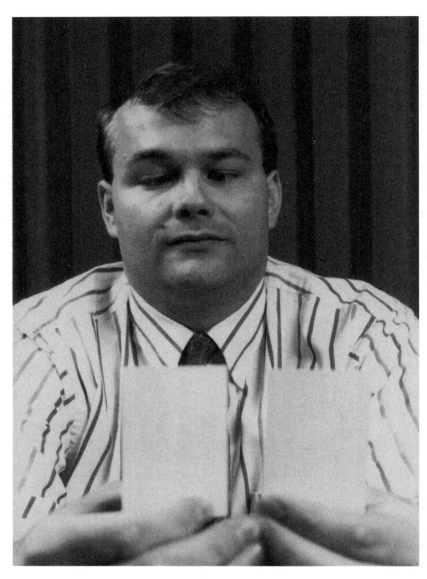

FIGURE 11.6
Training chiastopic fusion with Eccentric Circles on opaque cards.

The Keystone Colored Circles ("lifesavers") are separated to have increasing amounts of disparity from the bottom pair of circles on the card to the top pair; they are excellent for step vergence training. The two Eccentric Circle cards can be slowly separated to increase the disparity, which is excellent for sliding vergence training. The patient should be able to appreciate SILO effects and monitor for suppression while using these cards. Chiastopic and orthoptic fusion procedures, however, are often very difficult for children under 7 years of age.

The goal is to be able to achieve fusion quickly and clearly with increasing amounts of disparity. Further details on chiastopic and

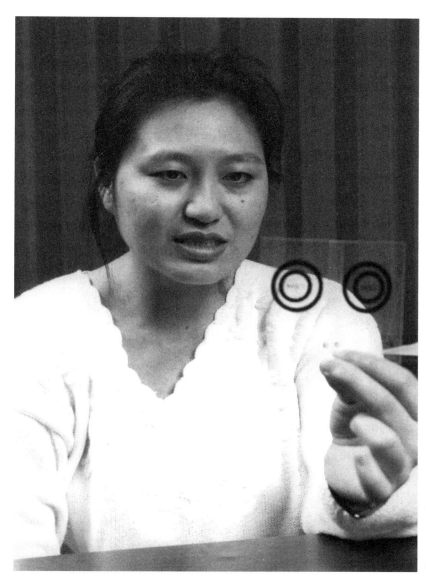

FIGURE 11.7
Training orthoptic fusion with eccentric circles on transparent cards.

orthoptic fusion training (and other VSE training techniques) are available in other sources.[1-4]

Visual-Perceptual-Motor Training Techniques

VPM therapy is organized into five parts: (1) bilateral integration, (2) laterality and directionality, (3) visual perception and visualization, (4) visual-motor integration, and (5) auditory-visual integration. As with VSE problems, deficiencies in these VPM functions can cause or contribute to RD. The clinician's training goal is for the patient to pass the testing criteria for each visual function (see Chapter 9) and to eliminate related symptoms and performance inefficiencies.

Bilateral Integration

Bilateral-integration therapy generally begins with gross motor activities and progresses to fine motor demands. Training in these activities should ensure good symmetric (opposite direction) and reciprocal (same direction) movements. During training, a metronome may be used and cognitive challenges may be added to help develop control and automaticity.

Steps in Bilateral-Integration Therapy

1. Develop the ability to conceptualize and execute a motor plan for gross bilateral integrative motor movements (this largely involves instilling in the patient a reflective rather than impulsive processing style).
2. Develop awareness of the two sides of the body (important for laterality therapy).
3. Develop auditory-visual integration in conjunction with a motor task.

Jumping Jacks

The exercise of performing jumping jacks can be used to train bilateral-integration skills. The patient is given instruction on how to perform a standard jumping jack: Start with feet together and arms at the sides, hop to move feet apart while simultaneously moving arms up, then hop to move feet back together and bring arms simultaneously back to the sides. This cycle should be repeated until it can be performed smoothly. A metronome is introduced to set the rhythm of the activity. The patient is instructed to move with each beat, that is, to move from the arms at sides and feet together position to arms above head and feet apart position. Variations on the positions of the arms and feet can be designed to challenge the patient further, such as starting with feet apart and arms at the sides and moving to feet together and arms up (Figure 11.8). The goal is to perform any variation of jumping jacks smoothly while integrating the movements to the beat of a metronome.

Windshield Wipers

This procedure develops symmetric and reciprocal bilateral integrative motor abilities. Two rectangles approximately 40 cm wide and 20 cm high are drawn on the chalkboard approximately 25 cm apart at the patient's eye level. A central fixation mark is drawn midway between the rectangles. The patient holds a piece of chalk in each hand, facing the fixation mark on the chalkboard, and places each chalk on the inner edge of each rectangle to start. Symmetric movements are trained first, in which the patient moves the chalk from the inner edge of the rectangles to the outer edge and back again while

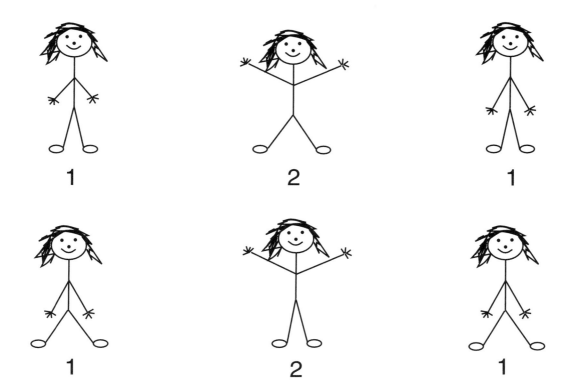

FIGURE 11.8 *Two patterns of jumping jacks.*

maintaining fixation on the central mark. These controlled, symmetric movements proceed from the midline of the body outward and then back toward the midline. Accuracy of marking from edge to edge is stressed. Reciprocal movements are trained in a similar manner: The patient starts with one chalk at the outer edge of one rectangle and the other chalk at the inner edge of the other rectangle (left-hand or right-hand edge). Both pieces of chalk are moved back and forth in the same direction, first left and then right. Be careful to avoid having the patient sway his or her entire body left and right; only the arms should move.

The goal is to be able to perform symmetric and reciprocal movements smoothly without loss of speed and position between the hands. Children under 7 years of age may not be able to perform accurate and quick reciprocal movements.

Laterality and Directionality

The sequence of therapy usually begins with laterality training (teaching the patient awareness of his or her own left and right sides) and proceeds to concepts of directionality (awareness of right and left sides of other people, animals, and objects). Ultimately, directionality for linguistic symbols should be achieved. When the patient masters knowledge of these concepts, automaticity can be developed by adding a metronome. Cognitive challenges can distract the patient from the task, and good automaticity is evident if the patient can continue to perform the training activity accurately while answering simple questions.

Steps in Laterality and Directionality Therapy

1. Develop the sense of left and right of the self (laterality).
2. Develop the sense of left and right of other people and objects (directionality).
3. Develop normal formation and recognition of correctly oriented numbers and letters.

Simon Says

The children's game of Simon Says is used to ask the patient to make laterality and directionality judgments. In this game, the therapist begins each command with "Simon says." If the command is not prefaced with "Simon says," the patient is not to perform the command, thus ensuring that the patient can pay attention to simple commands. Initially, laterality commands are given, such as "Simon says point to your left elbow." If appropriate for the age of the patient (generally by age 8 years), commands progress to directionality questions pertaining to the therapist, such as "Simon says point to my right knee."

When playing this game, it is important for the therapist to discuss with the patient strategies for making laterality and directionality judgments. The goal is to make correct judgments consistently.

Floor Map

This activity requires making a map on the floor, such as a masking tape trail with a series of right-angle turns. Training begins with laterality judgments. The patient is placed at the starting point of the map and instructed to direct himself through the turns by calling out the direction he must turn. It is sometimes helpful to have the patient signal with his arms which direction is indicated (for motor reinforcement). In the beginning of this therapy, the patient often guesses at the direction. In such cases, the therapist must help the patient to realize that one of his hands performs motor tasks better than the other, such as throwing a bean bag, writing one's name, and cutting with scissors. When the patient begins to understand this concept, the floor map training can be resumed. The therapist can remind the patient to figure out which is right and left by assigning a motor task, such as throwing a ball, to perform when there is difficulty with a directional judgment. With practice, the sense of the side with a motor advantage becomes more accessible to awareness, and further therapy will help make this skill more automatic.

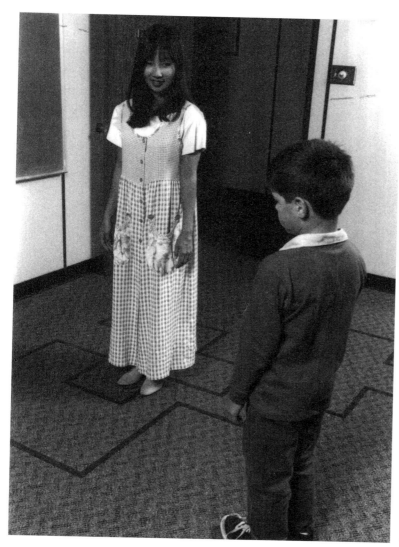

FIGURE 11.9   *Floor map with patient directing the therapist at each turn.*

When this level is mastered, the patient is asked to make directionality judgments by standing at the end of the map and guiding the therapist through it by calling out which direction the therapist must turn at each right angle (Figure 11.9). This is a difficult step, and the patient may initially need to turn his body to help make these judgments. This higher-level directionality is generally not appropriate for patients younger than 8 years old.

The goal is to perform each level with 100% accuracy. It is important to discuss strategies for making directional judgments at each level.

Directional Arrows

This activity is often referred to as Kirschner (a Canadian optometrist) arrows.[3] Training with directional arrows helps the patient develop

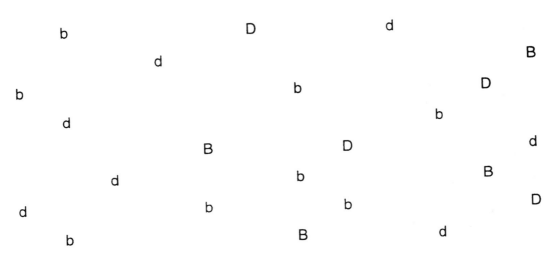

FIGURE 11.10   *A custom-made (computer-generated) letter find worksheet.*

directionality skills for printed symbols. An array of several rows of arrows is written on a chalkboard or a piece of paper with the arrows pointing up, down, left, or right in random order.

The patient is instructed to stand facing the arrows and to call out the direction of each arrow. The patient starts at the upper left corner and proceeds from left to right, row by row. Motor reinforcement can be provided by having the patient extend his or her arms out in front, placing hands together. As each arrow is fixated, the patient moves both arms in the same direction the arrow is pointing.

The goal is to call out each direction correctly with minimal hesitation. A metronome can be added to this task to increase automaticity. When the patient has mastered this task, he or she is instructed to call out the opposite direction of each arrow, pointing in either the same direction as the arrow or in the opposite direction. Such mismatches require exceptionally good directionality skills for successful performance.

Directionality for Numbers and Letters

Two levels of worksheets are used for training recognition of correct letter and number orientation. Such worksheets can be individually created. The first level requires the patient to identify specific letters in the correct orientation from an array of other letters, some of which are reversed. For the array shown in Figure 11.10, the patient might be asked to circle every lowercase *d* he or she finds. It is important to discuss how to differentiate the target letter from letters that are similar in appearance (e.g., *b* from *d*). Having the patient write the word *bed* is a prompt for *b* and *d* directionality, as the orthography resembles a bed with head and foot boards.

Cross out every backward letter you find.

dlue	hsll	doeɛ	bumq	bown
sonɡ	keǝp	poɳy	whγ	¡ust
rounb	pretʈy	ŧriend	garben	dehind
ɒlleɡiɒnce	elǝmentary	beceive	oqqosite

FIGURE 11.11 *A custom-made (computer-generated) worksheet for identification of reversed letters within words.*

The second level requires the patient to identify reversed letters within short words (Figure 11.11). It is important to use words within the eidetic decoding level of the patient. If the decoding level of the patient is known (e.g., from results of Dyslexia Determination Test), words of the appropriate level of difficulty are used for training purposes.

At each level, the goal is for the patient to achieve a high degree of accuracy (e.g., 90% correct responses with consistency). It is also important for the patient to be able to correct his or her own errors on the worksheets.

Visual Perception and Visualization

Many training activities can be used to improve motor-free visual perception. The therapist's role is to emphasize the patient's awareness of effective strategies necessary to perform the prescribed training tasks. Patients can then concentrate on strategies useful for development of the perceptual skill in question. For example, an individual who has difficulty with visual sequential memory may find that parsing the information (breaking the whole sequence into component parts) is an

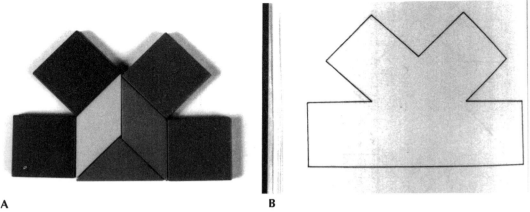

A   B

FIGURE 11.12   *Parquetry patterns requiring visual closure ability. With lines (A), and without lines (B) showing shapes of blocks necessary to complete the design.*

effective means of improving this type of memory. Ultimately, training of visualization skills should be emphasized; the patient must learn to manipulate visual information by cognitive means, such as remembering the sequence of a series of objects in reverse order.

Steps in Visual Perception and Visualization Therapy

1. Develop age-appropriate form perception, figure-ground, and visual closure abilities.
2. Develop the ability to create and recall images.
3. Develop sequential visual recall.
4. Develop visual image manipulation facility for problem solving.

Parquetry Blocks (Perceptual Emphasis)

Multicolored triangles, squares, and diamonds made of plastic or wood (parquetry) are used with workbooks containing line drawings composed of representations of the blocks (Figure 11.12). These blocks and designs can be created by the therapist. Parquetry block training can be used to develop visual discrimination, visual-spatial relationships, visual figure-ground, visual closure, visual memory, visual sequential memory, and visualization skills.

Beginning levels may contain designs consisting of only 2- to 5-block combinations. The patient must choose, from an assortment of blocks, the blocks necessary to recreate each design. To help a patient reproduce the designs, we recommend the following sequence: (1) the patient builds the design on top of the blocks the therapist used to build the design, (2) the patient builds the design next to the therapist's reproduction of the design, (3) the patient builds the design directly on top of the design printed on a workbook page, and (4) the patient builds the design to the side of the printed design of the workbook. When the patient has mastered step 4 with simple designs, more advanced designs are introduced. Steps 3 and 4 are repeated with designs that have no internal lines to identify which shapes are needed to complete the pattern. (Compare Figure 11.12A to 11.12B.) Visual memory and visual sequential memory abilities can be trained by allowing the patient to view the designs briefly before attempting to replicate the pattern. Visualization skills can be trained by asking the patient to reproduce the design as if it were rotated 90 degrees (a quarter turn) to the right or left. Goals to be achieved with parquetry blocks are individualized to the age and profile of each patient. Refer to Chapter 9, Visual-Perceptual-Motor Skills, for performance criteria.

Sequential Beads

This activity can be used to develop visual discrimination, visual-spatial relationships, visual figure-ground, visual sequential memory, and visualization abilities. A string of multicolored beads in a variety of shapes is needed for the procedure. Sets of beads, strings, and pattern cards can be designed by the therapist.

The patient is asked to reproduce designs shown on pattern cards created by the therapist. When the patient is able to replicate the designs easily, he or she is asked to remember the design and attempt to recreate it from memory. The number of beads needed to make each design should be gradually increased.

The goal for each patient is to be able to reproduce designs of appropriate length (based on age-expected performance) after only a brief look (5–10 seconds).

Tachistoscopic Activities (Numbers, Letters, Words)

A number of tachistoscopic devices and appropriate computer programs are commercially available (see the Appendix). These procedures can be used to develop visual sequential memory and visualization skills.

A series of printed symbols is briefly flashed (e.g., for 0.1 second) on a screen. Flash cards will suffice for home training. The patient must recall the sequence in the correct order. The sequence length is determined by reviewing the patient's performance on visual-perceptual evaluation (see Chapter 9, Visual-Perceptual-Motor Skills). Initially, numbers are used, then letters, and finally words, as the patient's skill improves. To add visualization demands to this task, the patient can be asked to reproduce the sequence in reverse of the order presented.

The goal is to recall correctly all the symbols flashed, most of the time. The patient should be encouraged to perform this task at very brief flash presentation times (e.g., 0.01 second).

Hidden Picture Games (Figures, Numbers, Letters, Words)

Many hidden picture workbooks are available wherever children's books and games are sold. These activities can develop visual discrimi-

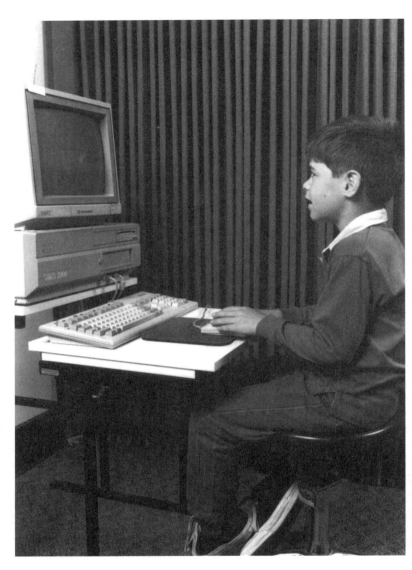

FIGURE 11.13
Patient performing vision therapy activities generated by a computer program (Opti-Mum[22]).

nation, visual-spatial relationships, visual form constancy, visual figure-ground, and visual memory skills.

The patient is shown a series of small objects that are embedded within a larger picture. The object can be oriented in any direction or be part of another object in the picture.

The goal is for the patient to be able to find the hidden objects easily in increasingly complex scenes.

Computerized Perceptual Games

Many commercially available computer programs contain activities designed to train VSE and VPM skills (Figure 11.13). Instructions are provided for the use of these programs when purchased. Most of the

TABLE 11.1A   Computer Orthoptics*

Program Name	Function
Visual Scan	VD, VFG, VM, saccades
Visual Sequential Processing	VSM
Tachistoscope	VSM, visualization, rapid visual processing
Visual Concentration	VM, VD, visualization
Visual Search	VSM, VD, saccades
Visual Span	VSM, auditory memory
Directionality	Visualization, directionality, VM
Visual Closure	VC, VFG, VD, visualization
Computer Pegboard	VSR, VFG, directionality, visualization

*Computerized vision therapy program available from RC Instruments, Cicero, IN.
VD = visual discrimination; VFG = visual figure-ground; VM = visual memory; VSM = visual sequential memory; VC = visual closure; VSR = visual-spatial relationships.

TABLE 11.1B   Opti-Mum*

Program Name	Function
Tachistoscope	VM, VD, visualization
Time-sequenced Objects	VSM, VD, auditory memory, visualization
Time-sequenced Groups	VSM, VD, auditory memory, visualization
Sames/Differences	VD, saccades
Tic-tac-toe	VM, VD, VSR, visualization
Space-sequenced Word Families	VD, language
Time-sequenced Word Families	Visualization, VD, VM, language
Sentence Identification	VM, visualization, language
Alphabet Jumbles	VD, VFG, saccades

*Computerized vision therapy program available from Learning Frontiers, Inc., Annapolis, MD.
VM = visual memory; VD = visual discrimination; VSM = visual sequential memory; VSR = visual-spatial relationships; VFG = visual figure-ground.

skill areas discussed in this chapter can be trained with these programs to a certain extent. Table 11.1 lists samples of Computer Orthoptics[21] and Opti-Mum[22] computerized vision therapy programs and some of the functions that can be trained with the programs. Maino[23] gave practical examples for the design of home-training worksheets, such as dive bombing and underlining x's and o's for saccadic eye movement training. Press[24] pointed out that, although many proprietary programs are available for computerized vision therapy, computer programs are intended to "complement rather than displace traditional therapy programs." The use of computers assists in motivating patients to perform therapy activities and provides quantitative performance information to the therapist. Duckman[25] advocated the application of computers in the management of functional and perceptual disorders in patients with developmental disabilities.

Golf Visualization

Simulated overhead views of a golf course are created on paper for this procedure. Visualization skills are developed as the patient attempts to play the course. The patient is asked to place the pencil tip on the first tee and form a mental blueprint of the design to the hole. With his or her eyes closed, the patient is asked to picture the blueprint and move the pencil, as though it were a golf ball, along the fairway toward the hole. When the patient thinks the tip of the pencil is in the hole, he or she can look to see where the tip of the pencil is. This is counted as one stroke. A stroke is necessarily added for every hazard, such as a sandtrap, that the pencil encounters. The patient must continue to close his or her eyes and try to get the tip of the pencil on the hole.

The patient's score for that hole is the total number of strokes counted to get to the hole. A score for the course can be calculated by adding together the total number of strokes for the course. The goal is to lower the patient's score for each course by using fewer strokes to get to each hole, indicating good visualization skill. We find that children as young as 7-years-old can grasp the concept of golfing. Other similar visualization games can be devised, however, if golfing is unfamiliar to the patient.

Flip Forms

Visualization procedures with flip forms can be performed on a chalkboard or with paper and pencil (Figure 11.14). The paper is divided into quarters with a cross drawn in the center, and a form is placed in the upper left quadrant (Figure 11.14A). The patient is instructed to imagine what that form would look like if it were flipped (rotated 90 degrees) around the vertical axis and then to draw the result in the upper right quadrant (Figure 11.14B). The patient is then asked to flip the form in the upper right quadrant around the horizontal axis and draw the result in the lower right quadrant (Figure 11.14C). The form in the lower right quadrant is then flipped around the vertical axis and drawn in the lower left quadrant (Figure 11.14D). The patient can check his or her accuracy by flipping the form in the lower left quadrant around the horizontal axis to see if it matches the original form in the upper left quadrant.

The goal of visualization is 100% accuracy when flipping increasingly complicated forms and to be able to identify mistakes and correct them.

Visual Coding Games

Visual coding games require the patient to use a decoder matrix to discover coded words. This training is to improve visualization and decoding of words. A matrix has numbers on one axis and letters on the other. At the intersection of each identifying number and letter is a letter. In Figure 11.15, for example, the letter *G* has the identifying

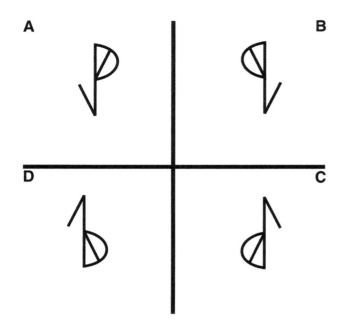

FIGURE 11.14 *Example of a flip form training procedure. A. Form in upper left corner shown to patient. B. Form in upper right corner drawn by patient, correctly "flipped" around the vertical axis. C. Form drawn by patient in the lower right corner, correctly flipped around the horizontal axis. D. Form drawn by patient in lower left corner, correctly flipped around the vertical axis.*

number-letter code of *D4* (the code describes the letter's position in the matrix). The patient is given a series of codes and asked what word is spelled by that code. For example, B5 + C1 + D4 spells *dog*. Later, the patient is not allowed to write down each letter as it is decoded but must keep the letters memorized until the whole word is spelled. The goal is to decode words of increasing length from progressively larger matrices.

Visual-Motor Integration

Therapy for visual-motor integration starts with manipulation of real objects and proceeds to replicating abstract representations with paper and pencil. The tasks are initially performed using highly structured designs to help guide the motoric responses. Eventually, the same replication tasks are made more difficult by using designs with less structure.

Steps in Visual-Motor Integration Therapy

1. Develop the ability to make visual distance and size judgments.
2. Develop an organized approach to visual-motor tasks (e.g., top to bottom and left to right).
3. Develop a projective (motor planning) visual-motor style rather than a bit-by-bit (stimulus-bound) style.
4. Develop a spatial coordinate system for visual-motor tasks and for visual closure.
5. Develop speed, accuracy, and facility for academic paper and pencil tasks.

	1	2	3	4	5
A	T	A	M	Y	F
B	B	R	I	L	D
C	O	P	C	K	H
D	E	S	N	G	U

___ ___ ___
B 5   C 1   D 4

___ ___ ___ ___
D 4   B 3   B 2   B 4

___ ___ ___ ___ ___
C 5   C 1   D 5   D 2   D 1

___ ___ ___ ___ ___ ___
C 3   A 2   A 1   D 3   A 2   C 2

FIGURE 11.15 *A custom-made visual decoding game.*

Spatial Relations

The patient is presented with a spatial problem, such as judging how many paces are required to walk across the room. This can be done with the patient standing with his or her back to one wall. Length, width, and diagonal distances can be assessed to see if the child generally understands the relation between these various dimensions. When the child consistently estimates distances to within one or two paces, he or she should be asked to estimate half the distances.

Rosner Program

The Rosner program is an extension of the test for visual analysis skills (TVAS).[26] This program has up to 200 line patterns that are produced

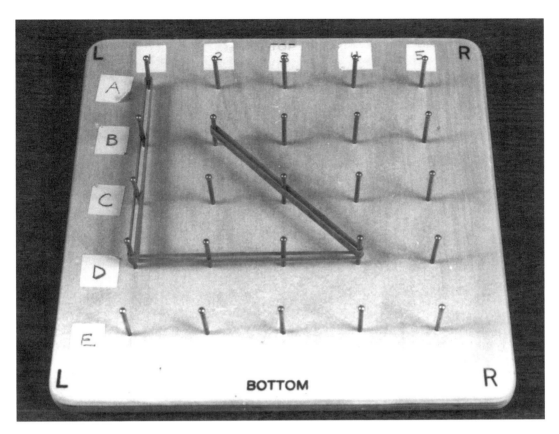

FIGURE 11.16   *Geoboard for visual-motor integration training.*

on dotted grids made of 5–25 evenly spaced dots. These lined patterns are to be copied with a pencil onto other grids, either dotted or on blank paper, to develop vision-directed fine motor planning and execution. Initially, a geoboard (a wooden square with a grid of nails) can be used to copy the first 150 patterns with rubber bands (Figure 11.16). Many training variations are possible. In one variation, the therapist strings rubber bands to replicate a Rosner lined pattern. The patient puts rubber bands on top of the pattern for a superimposed replication. Next, the patient can construct a pattern of the therapist's geoboard on his or her own geoboard adjacent to that of the therapist. Finally, the patient can construct the lined patterns from a printed worksheet onto the geoboard. It is suggested that the TVAS be administered prior to training to determine an appropriate beginning level.

For advanced training without a geoboard, a worksheet of dotted grids is placed in front of the patient. The pattern to be reproduced is drawn by the therapist on one of the blank grids. The patient is asked to copy the pattern on another grid next to the one with the pattern. During the copying process, it is important to ask the patient to verbalize his or her strategy for determining where to draw each line on the grid. Development of appropriate analysis of a pattern and planning of its reproduction is crucial in the training process. This training technique, therefore, also develops visual-perception and visualization skills. The patient is asked to copy progressively more complex patterns without having the therapist copy the patterns first. This is repeated until the patient has mastered the ability to copy the patterns onto 25-dot grids. The patient is then asked to copy the same complex patterns (150–200) onto grids with progressively fewer dots (e.g., 17-, 9-, 5-, and 0-dot grids). The goal is to reproduce the complex patterns neatly without erasing and with the structure of a dot grid.

Ideal Forms

Ideal Forms for visual-motor integration training are a set of worksheets designed to provide progressively difficult forms to be reproduced (see the Appendix). These forms are to be copied with a pencil to develop vision-directed, fine-motor planning and execution (Figure 11.17).

Each row of the Ideal Forms contains four squares. The first square on the left contains the shape to be replicated. The second square contains the same shape as the first square, but the lines are incomplete. The patient is asked to trace over the incomplete lines, thereby completing the shape. The third square is blank, and the patient is asked to replicate the shape in this square. The last square is also blank, and the patient is asked to draw the shape again with the first three squares covered. The last task requires visual memory in addition to good visual-motor integration skills. The patient progresses through the increasingly difficult shapes with continuing encouragement to self-monitor each drawing for accuracy. The ultimate goal is to accurately copy from memory each shape in the fourth square without looking at the original figure in the first square.

Auditory-Visual Integration

Therapy for auditory-visual integration usually begins with nonlinguistic auditory (e.g., tapping sounds) and visual (e.g., printed dots) stimuli. Training progresses to the use of oral and written stimuli (letters and words) commensurate with decoding levels of the Dyslexia Determination Test. It is important to ensure that patients have developed good visual and auditory memory as well as visualization skills before training of auditory-visual integration skills. This is particularly necessary when therapy involves decoding and encoding of words.

Steps in Auditory-Visual Integration Therapy

1. Develop the ability to discriminate and remember auditory stimuli.
2. Develop awareness of the relation between auditory patterns and a visual-spatial representation of them.

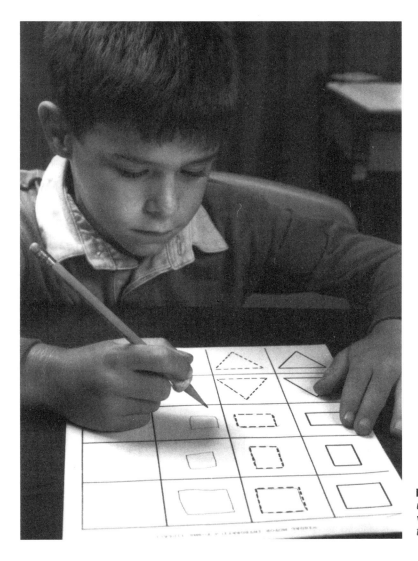

FIGURE 11.17 *Patient using Ideal Forms for visual-motor integration training.*

3. Develop the awareness that written language involves symbols that stand for various sounds that, when taken together, form words.

Clap Patterns

This therapy procedure can be used to improve auditory discrimination, auditory-visual integration, auditory-sequential memory, and visualization. It is excellent for children under 8 years of age.[27] The patient is instructed to listen (without looking) to various clap patterns produced by the therapist. For example, with clap-pause-clap-clap and clap-clap-pause-clap patterns, the patient is asked whether the patterns were the same or different. Also, the child can be instructed to watch, listen, and replicate the clapping pattern produced by the therapist.

The goal is to replicate patterns of increasing length (refer to the auditory-visual integration test in Chapter 9 to help match the patient's ability with the developmental norms for his or her age). The patient can also be asked to spell a word while repeating the pattern (one letter for each clap).

Computerized Auditory Games

Many computer programs feature activities that can be used to train auditory-visual integration, as well as auditory-sequential memory and visualization skills. For example, on the Opti-Mum system, the Time-sequenced Objects program can be used. The patient is instructed to face away from the computer screen and listen to the naming of a series of objects sounded by the computer. The computer may, for example, display and name the following sequence: bee, flower, square, house. The patient then looks at the computer keyboard and responds by pressing the corresponding function keys. This serves as feedback for accuracy. Visualization skills can be trained by asking the patient to repeat the series in the reverse order of presentation. The goal is to achieve a high level of accuracy in repeating sequences of age-appropriate length.

Morse Code (Decoding and Encoding)

Teaching a patient how to listen to and interpret Morse code signals trains in high levels of auditory discrimination, auditory sequential memory, and visualization. The patient is given a Morse code key (Figure 11.18) to learn, then letters are signaled (via dots and dashes) individually to assist the patient in interpreting the signals. This technique is for older children and adults. To train sequential memory and visualization, single letters are signaled to form a word. The patient must listen and interpret each letter, then write the word when it is completed. The goal is to decode, with a high level of accuracy, words and messages of increasing length.

Summary

Optometric therapy is often effective in eliminating contributory vision problems in RD. Vision therapy can improve the visual efficiency skills of saccades, accommodation, vergence, and VPM skills of bilateral integration, laterality and directionality, visual perception and visualization, visual-motor integration, and auditory-visual integration. All these pertinent skills should be treated, when necessary, in patients with RD.

A	• —
B	— • • •
C	— • — •
D	— • •
E	•
F	• • — •
G	— — •
H	• • • •
I	• •
J	• — — —
K	— • —
L	• — • •
M	— —
N	— •
O	— — —
P	• — — •
Q	— — • —
R	• — •
S	• • •
T	—
U	• • —
V	• • • —
W	• — —
X	— • • —
Y	— • — —
Z	— — • •
1	• — — — —
2	• • — — —
3	• • • — —
4	• • • • —
5	• • • • •
6	— • • • •
7	— — • • •
8	— — — • •
9	— — — — •
0	— — — — —
Period	• — • — • —
Comma	— — • • — —
Colon	— — — • • •
Query	• • — — • •
Apostrophe	• — — — — •
Hyphen	— • • • • —
Fraction Bar	— • • — •
Parentheses	— • — — • —
Quotation Marks	• — • • — •

FIGURE 11.18 *Key for the Morse code.*

References

1. Griffin JR, Grisham JD. Binocular Anomalies: Diagnosis and Vision Therapy (3rd ed). Boston: Butterworth-Heinemann, 1995.
2. Birnbaum MH. Optometric Management of Nearpoint Vision Disorders. Boston: Butterworth-Heinemann, 1993.
3. Scheiman MM, Rouse MW. Optometric Management of Learning-Related Vision Problems. Boston: Butterworth-Heinemann, 1994.
4. Scheiman M, Wick B. Clinical Management of Binocular Vision: Heterophoric, Accommodative, and Eye Movement Disorders. Philadelphia: Lippincott, 1994.
5. Cohen AH (1986/87 Task Force). The efficacy of optometric vision therapy. J Am Optom Assoc 1988;59:95–105.
6. Solan HA, Mozlin R. The correlations of perceptual-motor maturation to readiness and reading in kindergarten and the primary grades. J Am Optom Assoc 1986;57:28–35.
7. Garzia RP, Nicholson SB. Visual function and reading disability: an optometric viewpoint. J Am Optom Assoc 1990;61:88–97.
8. Lovegrove WJ, Garzia RP. Experimental evidence for a transient deficit in specific reading disability. J Am Optom Assoc 1990;61:137–46.
9. Williams MC, Lecluyse K. Perceptual consequences of a temporal processing deficit in reading disabled children. J Am Optom Assoc 1990;61:111–21.
10. Garzia RP, Sesma M. Vision and reading: neuroanatomy and electrophysiology. J Optom Vis Dev 1993;24:4–51.
11. Borsting E, Ridder WH, Dudeck K, et al. The presence of a magnocellular defect depends on the type of dyslexia. Vision Res 1996;36:1047–53.
12. Galaburda AM. The Pathogenesis of Childhood Dyslexia. In F Plum (ed), Brain. New York: Raven, 1988.
13. Solan HA. Transient and sustained processing: a dual subsystem theory of reading disability. J Behav Optom 1994;5:149–54.
14. Scheiman M, Blaskey P, Ciner E, et al. Vision characteristics of individuals identified as Irlen filter candidates. J Am Optom Assoc 1990;61:600–5.
15. Cardinal DN, Griffin JR, Christenson GN. Do tinted lenses really help students with reading disabilities? Intervention School Clin 1993;28:275–9.
16. Mesulam MM. A cortical network for directed attention and unilateral neglect. Ann Neurol 1981;10:309–25.
17. Warren M. Evaluation and treatment of visual perceptual dysfunction in acute brain injury. Presented at St. Cloud State University, MN, February 1993.
18. Gibson KH, Gibson KD. Visual processing therapy and changes in higher cognitive abilities. (Gulf Breeze, Fl) 1996 (submitted).
19. Birnbaum MH. Behavioral optometry: a historical perspective. J Am Optom Assoc 1994;65:255–64.
20. Cool S. Viewpoint: behavioral optometry and occupational therapy: an interactive whose time has come. J Behav Optom 1990;1:31–2.
21. Computer Orthoptics (computerized vision therapy program). RC Instruments, 99 West Jackson Street, Cicero, IN 46034.
22. Opti-Mum (computerized vision therapy program). Learning Frontiers, Inc. 190 Admiral Cochran Dr., Suite 180, Annapolis, MD 21401.

23. Maino DM. Applications in Pediatrics, Binocular Vision, and Perception. In JH Maino, DM Maino, DW Davison (eds), Computer Applications in Optometry. Boston: Butterworth, 1989;99–122.
24. Press LJ, Moore BD. Clinical Pediatric Optometry. Boston: Butterworth-Heinemann, 1993;325.
25. Duckman RH. Management of Functional and Perceptual Disorders in Patients with Developmental Disabilities. In DM Maino (ed), Diagnosis and Management of Special Populations. St. Louis: Mosby 1995;256–63.
26. Rosner J. Helping Children Overcome Learning Difficulties (3rd ed). New York: Walker, 1993.
27. Erickson GB, Griffin JR. Thinking goes to vision therapy. J Behav Optom 1993;4:115–7.

12 Optometric Management and the Multidisciplinary Approach

Optometric management of reading dysfunction (RD) often requires a multidisciplinary approach. The role of the optometrist includes diagnosis and treatment of binocular and perceptual skills, which include visual skills efficiency (VSE) and visual-perceptual-motor (VPM) skills; assessment of dyslexia; and recommendations for appropriate therapy. Case studies are presented to clarify clinical applications of optometric management.

General Reading Dysfunction

An individual with general RD may have such contributory causes as low intelligence; educational deprivation; bilingual confusion; vision, auditory, or sensory integration problems; or attentional problems, as well as other problems of various etiologies. When all these possible causes are ruled out, the RD is traditionally presumed due to dyslexia. Direct diagnostic testing for dyslexia becomes very important.

Optometric Role in General Reading Dysfunction

Christenson et al.[1] discussed the role of the optometrist in detail. If dyslexia testing rules out dyslexia, and the nonvisual causes of RD are ruled out by a school psychologist or a resource specialist, the optometrist should conduct a thorough evaluation of VSE and VPM skills. If any vision problems are found that could partially or wholly account for the RD, optometric vision therapy should be recommended.

Referral Recommendations

If the optometrist is a primary eye care practitioner not specializing in vision therapy, a referral should be made to an optometric specialist who can provide further assessment and appropriate vision therapy (if needed) for the patient with general RD. Referral for educational assessment is frequently recommended. The optometrist, either the primary or specialty practitioner, is often the coordinator of the multidisciplinary team. Unless there is a team working together to benefit an individual with RD, effective therapy may be delayed or even entirely forsaken. Along with referral to an education specialist, the optometrist should refer the patient, if necessary, to a physician, psychologist, occupational therapist, or other professionals as called for in each particular case.

The optometrist can comanage a case of general RD by ensuring that all vision-related reading problems are diagnosed and treated, when feasible. Communication with all members of the multidisciplinary team should continue because follow-up visits will be scheduled. The goal for the optometrist and other professionals on the team is to ensure that all contributory causes are eliminated (when possible) so that the general RD may be resolved.

Specific Reading Dysfunction (Dyslexia)

As stated previously, the optometrist should determine whether the RD is general or specific. The optometrist's role in cases of dyslexia is similar to that in general RD, but greater emphasis is placed on referral for educational therapy.

TABLE 12.1   General Guidelines for Prognosis in Dyslexia

Type and Severity	Therapeutic Approach	Eventual Goal of Therapy	Predicted Success
Dysnemkinesia, mild	Optometric vision therapy for laterality and direction-ality skills; aspects may be included in educational therapy	Elimination of number and letter reversals by 5th grade	90%
Dysnemkinesia, marked	Same	Elimination by 7th grade	85%
Dysphonesia, mild	Educational therapy with initial emphasis on look-say (ei-detic) decoding skills; later, phonetic training	Improved eidetic skills enable reading almost to expected grade level; decoding of unfamiliar words improved but not completely normal	80%
Dysphonesia, marked	Same	Lower-division college reading level at best; otherwise, same as mild dysphonesia	75%
Dyseidesia, mild	Educational therapy with train-ing in phonics; when phon-etic skills are mastered, look-say eidetic training can be given	Develop normal phonetic de-coding and encoding skills; reading level 12th grade at best; minor spelling prob-lems remain, with reliance on phonetic equivalents	70%
Dyseidesia, marked	Same as for mild dyseidesia but with intense educational therapy	10th-grade reading level at best; increased spelling errors remain with great reliance on phonetic equivalents	65%
Dysphoneidesia, mild	Educational therapy with in-tense multisensory and written-language training, including phonetic and ei-detic approaches coordi-nated with continuing tactile-kinesthetic activities	8th-grade reading level at best; major spelling errors remain, with poor eidetic and phon-etic encoding; if dysphonetic component can be abated, the reading level may be higher	60%
Dysphoneidesia, marked	Same as for mild dysphonei-desia, but more intense edu-cational therapy required	6th-grade reading level at best; major spelling problems	55%

Optometric Role in Specific Reading Dysfunction

At the heart of multidisciplinary treatment of dyslexia is the need for understanding dyslexia and its diagnosis, prognosis, and treatment (Table 12.1). Aside from the previously mentioned health professionals involved in the field of RD, nurses may be involved as important screeners for dyslexia, particularly in school-aged children. All health professionals should coordinate with education professionals.[1,2] Dyslexia screening and testing can begin at the kindergarten level.

TABLE 12.2   Screening for Dyslexia by the Optometrist

Informal screening

Decoding is assessed by having the patient read aloud a paragraph from a text appropriate to his or her grade in school. The optometrist listens for missed words and notes whether reading is slow. If reading is slow and inaccurate, a new paragraph is read to the patient and content questions asked. If questions can be answered appropriately, comprehension is normal. If this is so when word decoding is slow or inaccurate, suspect dyslexia.

Ask the patient to write the answers. Poor encoding is indicated by spelling errors (either dyseidesia or dysphonesia).

Ask the patient to print some answers. Too many reversals indicate dysnemkinesia (e.g., a third-grade student should have few, if any, letter reversals).

Formal screening

The Dyslexia Screener can be used. Dyseidesia is indicated if eidetic decoding is lower than expected for grade placement and if encoding reveals poor visual memory for words (e.g., *duz* for *does*).

Dysphonesia is indicated by poor phonetic encoding (e.g., *dose* for *does*).

The Dyslexia Determination Test can be used for formal testing of dysnemkinesia.

Optometric vision therapy must be commensurate with patients' particular abilities as to age expectancies, based on the results of tests such as those discussed in Chapter 9.

Screening for Dyslexia

Careful case history is the first step in screening for dyslexia.[3] Reports of slow reading or poor writing and spelling indicate the need for screening. This can first be done informally (Table 12.2 and Figure 12.1). Suspected decoding and encoding problems turned up by informal screening indicate the need for further investigation with The Dyslexia Screener (TDS)[4] or possibly formal testing (see Chapter 10). Christenson et al.[5] established the validity of TDS, and Guerin et al.[6] showed the validity of mass screening by comparing the TDS with the Woodcock-Johnson Psychoeducational Assessment Battery. Formal screening for dysnemkinesia can be done with the Dyslexia Determination Test (DDT).[7]

For patients in kindergarten, the Predyslexia Letter Coding Test (PLCT)[8] can be used for predictive screening of dyslexia. First-grade students can be screened with the Dyslexia Screener for First-graders (DSF).[9] Adults suspected of having dyslexia can be tested with the Adult Dyslexia Test (ADT).[10] The ADT was evaluated by Biberdorf et al.[11] in a sample of college students. Their results supported the use of ADT in optometric practice. Spanish and French (Canadian) speakers can be tested with foreign-language versions of the DDT.[12, 13]

Prognosis in Dyslexia

The prognosis is based on professional judgment. The treatment goal is to improve reading ability to the individual's maximum ability. General guidelines for prognosis based on our clinical experience are shown in

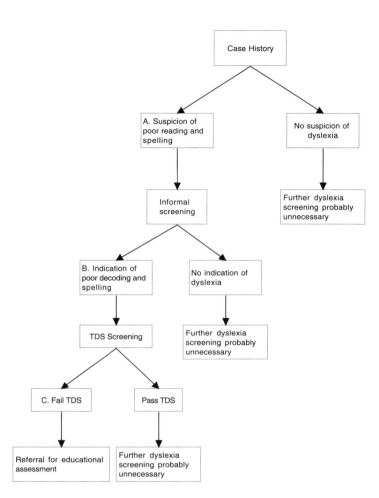

FIGURE 12.1 *Office screening for dyslexia. A. Patient has a history of poor reading and spelling. B. Read to patient followed by questions (see Table 12.2). C. Borderline or worse suggests referral. (TDS = The Dyslexia Screener.)*

Table 12.1. We have found that patients with marked dysphoneidesia, for example, are rarely able to achieve a reading level much above the sixth grade, assuming average intelligence and otherwise normal conditions. This apparent limitation of reading, however, does not mean these individuals are precluded from their vocational and avocational goals. Case examples presented later in the chapter illustrate achievement possibilities in dyslexic individuals.

Referral for Educational Therapy

The optometrist should consider referring all patients with dyslexia for educational testing and assessment of RD. The following topics are discussed with regard to educational therapy: trends, importance of early diagnosis, special education placement, approaches to teaching reading, and efficacy of multidisciplinary therapy.

Trends in Educational Policy

The basis for educational assessment and placement of reading disabled students is Public Law (PL) 94-142, the Education for All Handicapped Act of 1975.[14] The law requires handicapped children to be educated in the least restrictive environment possible. Each handicapped child should have an individualized educational plan (IEP) that details the steps of instruction leading to an educational environment that is as integrated with nonhandicapped students as possible. The IEP is to be rewritten each year and should include educational goals and methods for achievement. Parents have the right to have the plan reviewed periodically and updated or changed. Details are worked out with the school's multidisciplinary team to comply with the parent's wishes and the resources of the school. In learning disability, including RD, a psychoeducational evaluation must be performed to determine if the child qualifies for special education services under PL 94-142. This evaluation involves intelligence and achievement testing to find out if a significant disparity between intelligence and achievement exists. Generally, a 2-year disparity is required for the child to qualify for special education. Once the child qualifies, an IEP is written and special educational services are implemented.

PL 94-142 indicated the need for assessment by an optometrist of visual skills functioning. According to Lemer,[14] visual-perceptual problems could also be confirmed by the optometrist in a child suspected of having a specific learning disability. Subsequently, "If the optometric diagnosis confirms a perceptual handicap, the learning-disabled child may then receive appropriate services." This implies authorization of VPM therapy. More certainly, the law provides that "related services" be provided. "Consequently, patients with oculomotor, binocular, and accommodative dysfunctions, which impede the acquisition of academic skills, can thus receive optometric services under the law." Unfortunately, receiving authorization from the school district can be a lengthy process; timely treatment should be funded by other means (e.g., major medical benefits or sliding-scale fee agreements).

Subsequent legislation to the 1975 law was the Individuals with Disability Education Act of 1993.[15] It stated provisions to include "the related services necessary for the child to benefit from the classroom program in the least restricted educational environment." This particular inclusion has led to the trend of "mainstreaming" special education students into the regular classroom.

This system has two main drawbacks. First, it requires the student to have "failed" for at least 2 years before any intervention can be attempted, which can have devastating effects on the child's self-esteem. Second, many schools are not equipped to handle the special needs of all children with specific RD. Some children remain in the regular classroom, where they do not have the skills to compete successfully. A practical solution to these shortcomings can be sought by providing an understanding by all members of the IEP team of the nature of the RD, particularly when it is due to dyslexia.

Pertinent trends in education are (1) referral of problem students for attention-deficit hyperactivity disorder (ADHD), (2) movement toward full inclusion for all students with learning disabilities, and (3) implementation of a strict whole-language curriculum for reading instruction.

ADHD is often diagnosed subjectively based on observation of the child and questioning of the parents and teacher. Based on these impressions, medication (e.g., methylphenidate [Ritalin], pemoline [Cylert], dextroamphetamine [Dexedrine]) may be prescribed. If the child's subsequent activity level is thought to be too subdued, the medication is reduced and re-evaluated until the optimal dosage is achieved. The subjective nature of this diagnosis and treatment leaves the ADHD label open to criticism. We have comanaged some cases in which medication greatly benefited the child. Our concern, however, is the frequent prescription of medication for children struggling with reading, spelling, and writing. Referral is often made with little or no attempt to test directly for dyslexia (e.g., with DDT) to discover whether it is a factor in the child's academic difficulty. The practical problem of lack of special services in the public schools intensifies this dilemma. Teachers and administrators are put in the position of wanting and needing to do something. Regrettably, it is possible that many children are over-referred for medication to treat ADHD.

A recently introduced test for attention disorders by Universal Attention Disorders, Inc. (see the Appendix) is the Test of Variable Attention (TOVA). This test is compatible with various computers. The TOVA program has a duration of 22.5 minutes so that shorter attention spans can be detected. This test is applicable for ages 4–80 and up. Testing time for 4- and 5-year-olds, however, is reduced to 11.5 minutes. Image stimuli consist of a large square containing a smaller square adjacent to either the top or bottom edge of the larger square. The smaller square is intermittently presented for 100 milliseconds every 2 seconds. The smaller top square is the designated target to which the patient is asked to respond when displayed on the video screen. Test results are scored and ranked by computer to assess errors of omission and commission as well as response times and variability. Established norms are used to differentiate normal responders from those with attention-deficit disorder. Computerized controlled testing procedures may be helpful for reliable ADHD diagnosing, which may address the issue of over-referral for medication.

The trend of full inclusion creates obstacles to the child with dyslexia. *Full inclusion* means the same placement, instruction, and treatment for all students with learning disabilities as students in the regular classroom. A group called Learning Disabilities of America (LDA) does not fully support this trend. LDA feels that many students with learning disabilities benefit from being in the regular classroom, but it is not the appropriate placement for a number of students with learning disabilities who may need alternative instructional environments, teaching strategies, and materials not provided in regular classrooms.

Another trend, whole-language instruction, is a literature-based instructional approach predicated on the premise that immersing a student in the cognitive experience of reading will motivate him or her to learn to read. This method, the ultimate top-down approach, neglects the decoding needs of a child with dyslexia. Wilson[16] addresses the problem presented by the whole-language approach: "If a student has not successfully learned to read and is in middle (junior high) school or high school, that student will achieve poorly in a regular English class studying literature." Studying literature is a critical part of every student's curriculum, but students must also become independent readers, which may be difficult for students with dyslexia.

Importance of Early Diagnosis of Dyslexia

The core issue of the educational needs of a child with RD revolves around early diagnosis. Under the present system in many schools, a child must be 2 years behind in reading before being considered for special services. Children pay a high emotional price as they continually fail at academic tasks while waiting to qualify for help.[17]

Many educators seem to have a limited understanding of the biology, genetics, and fundamental nature of dyslexia. This is not to denigrate pioneers in the field, but rather to say that leaps in understanding have been made. It is time to apply this knowledge at a practical level by ensuring early identification of children with RD. Direct identification can be done as early as kindergarten.

The PLCT, DSF, and TDS allow for screening in the early grades. A dyslexic RD, or a predisposition for it, can be detected before the child experiences the adverse effects of failure. Appropriate educational strategies and treatment can then be implemented. Note that the authors of this text are some of the coauthors of these tests; research and clinical experience led to the development of these assessment tools.

An example of an integrated approach is found at the New Visions School in Minneapolis. This charter school is designed to meet the needs of children with RD. Principles of intervention include early identification and multidisciplinary services for development of fundamental skills, such as optometric vision therapy and occupational therapy. Educational principles are centered in multisensory, structured, phonetic training to ground students in the logic and structure of written language (reading, writing, and spelling). It is understandable that few public schools are equipped to function as a charter school expressly designed to help students with RD. Nevertheless, these applications can be helpful in regular classrooms of public schools.

It is time to recognize that a single method of language instruction is not appropriate for all children. Teachers, administrators, and affiliated personnel working in the public school system must understand that some children with normal intelligence require the multisensory phonetic approach when learning to read and spell. It is true that many nondyslexic children learn to read very efficiently with the whole-language approach and that, in this advanced group, the multisensory phonetic training may be boring, cumbersome, and unnecessary. The key to differentiating the two groups lies in an understanding of dyslexia. There are fundamental differences in the processing of the symbols of written language between children with dyslexia and nondyslexic good readers. When all members of the educational team understand these differences, it is not difficult to devise programs to meet the needs of children with dyslexia. The process starts with proper identification of the type and severity of the RD. Decisions can then be made for the type of intervention required. In cases of mild dyslexia, the problem may often be dealt with in the regular classroom when intervention occurs in the early grades. The teacher may divide the class into two sections and use a literature-based approach with one group and a multisensory approach with the other. Alternatively, the teacher may blend the whole-language approach and the multisensory, phonetic strategy to the benefit of all students. In other settings, an aide may be used to work with one group. All these solutions require a teacher with a thorough understanding of RD, who is well versed in the various methods of instruction.

In more severe cases of dyslexia, services beyond the scope of the regular classroom are required; placement in special education schools becomes necessary. This brings us to the point of reforming the manner in which children qualify for placement in learning disability programs.

Facilitating Special Education Placement

We believe that it is time to institute a new system of determining who needs special intervention for RD. It is clear that RD must be identified early and intervention begun in the regular classroom. Further discussion must address direct diagnosis for placement versus the present system of exclusionary diagnosis alone. Our knowledge has evolved to the point at which dyslexia can be diagnosed directly, and this process should be central to the determination of placement in special education. The issue of placement for RD should start with direct dyslexia testing. Criteria such as the type and severity of the dyslexia and the disparity between reading level and intelligence can then be considered in placement decisions. For students whose dyslexia has caused them to fall far behind, an intense course of multisensory phonetic training and other multidisciplinary professional services will likely be required.

Educational and Multisensory Approaches

We have discussed the scientific foundation and clinical application of vision therapy in cases of RD. We present an overview of the principles of a structured, multisensory, phonetically based language therapy program. This recommended educational approach (and many similar ones) is based on the traditional method of written language instruction, referred to as *Orton-Gillingham.*

Whole-Language Approach

Debate continues on how reading skills should be taught. This issue is important because many children struggle to learn to read. We surmise that many of these struggling students are dyslexic. Proponents of the whole-language approach have gained support in recent years. Unfortunately, in many schools, little or no time is spent on drilling basic written language concepts, such as phonetics, syllabication, and affixes. The whole-language approach does not emphasize decoding and encoding or many other important aspects of the structure and logic of written language. Instead, emphasis is supposed to be on the global literary experience of reading and fostering the learning process by capturing the child's imagination through the use of motivationally relevant materials and creating an environment in which the student wants to read. All of these goals are important, but without learning the structure of the written language code, some students will have great difficulty learning to read. Many educators have become opponents of the strict whole-language movement. One reason is that reading levels of students in many schools have fallen since the advent of the whole-language approach. Many of these opponents, however, also need to recognize the neurologic and behavioral aspects of dyslexia.

Phonetic Approach

Teachers generally recognize the phonetic approach to written language instruction as the most sensible approach to help delayed readers, and research supports this contention. Phonologic awareness, the recognition that words are made up of discrete units, is the best single predictor of reading achievement.[18–24] This lets the beginning reader *know* that words can be spelled even though spelling skills remain to be developed. The development of phonetic skills is critical in teaching delayed readers.[25–29] Phonologic awareness is related to auditory-visual integration (see Chapter 9); Solan and Mozlin[30] found that this correlated highly with reading achievement in the early grades. In optometric vision therapy auditory-visual integration often plays an important part in the treatment of RD.

The phonologic approach contrasts with the whole-language philosophy, which is founded on the assumption that learning to read and write is a natural extension of listening and speaking, and there is little or no need for training symbol-sound relationships. The whole-language approach promotes attainment of a sight-word lexicon by learning to guess at new words based on context and prior knowledge. This is encouraged by immersing the child in the experience of reading and writing through storytelling and motivating the student to

TABLE 12.3   General Pronunciation Rules for Short Vowel Sounds

Letter	Example
a	bat
e	bed
i	bid
o	not
u	cup

be interested in gaining knowledge through the printed word. This method may help above-normal readers, but we believe that an exclusively whole-language approach is a ticket to failure for the dyslexic child.

Optometrists are not expected to have extensive knowledge of phonics. (*Phonics* refers to the use of phonetic teaching in reading; *phonetics* refers to the representation of speech sounds with written symbols, namely, the letters of the alphabet.) Our purpose here is to introduce the phonetic application in education so that the optometric practitioner can have a basic understanding of some phonetic principles and appreciate its importance in the learning-to-read process.

Teaching of phonetic decoding begins with matching letters of the alphabet with their names and sounds. For example, *b* has the sound *buh* rather than *bee*, as it is named. The PLCT provides testing of letter decoding and further explanations.[8] Most consonants in the English language have a unitary match, meaning that the letter sound does not change from word to word. Notable exceptions are the letters *c* and *g*. The letter *c* acts as though it were a *k* when it comes before the letters *a, o,* or *u,* as in *cat, cot,* and *cut. C* has the sound of *s* before the letters *e, i,* and *y,* as in *cent, city,* and *cycle.*

Unlike consonants, vowels have many sounds. Tables 12.3 and 12.4 show how a single letter sound varies in different words. Many other rules of phonics pertain to syllables and words. Numerous books, videos, and computer programs teach phonetic rules (Table 12.5). Along with phonetic rules, the dyslexic individual requires multisensory written language instruction.

Multisensory Language Approach

Multisensory, phonetic, written-language instruction usually involves a student-teacher ratio of no more than 4 to 1. At the New Visions School in Minneapolis, students are grouped according to ability levels based on preliminary assessment of their familiarity with symbol-sound relationships and the rules of written language. More than 100 sounds and the rules that apply to their usage in words must be mastered. The sounds are subdivided into categories that are organized for ease of instruction during teaching sessions (Figure 12.2).

TABLE 12.4   General Pronunciation Rules for Long Vowel Sounds

Letter	Rule	Example
a	marker e	can and c<u>a</u>ne
a	a before i	p<u>ai</u>n
a	a before y	d<u>ay</u>
e	e before a	<u>ea</u>t
e	e before e	s<u>ee</u>
e	e before y	k<u>ey</u>
i	marker e	hid and h<u>i</u>de
i	i before e	p<u>ie</u>
i	i before gh	l<u>igh</u>t
o	marker e	not and n<u>o</u>te
o	o before a	b<u>oa</u>t
o	o before e	t<u>oe</u>
o	o before w	l<u>ow</u>
o	ending o (word or possibly syllable)	n<u>o</u>, pol<u>o</u>
u	marker e	cut and c<u>u</u>te
u	u before i	j<u>ui</u>ce
y	The letter y may sound as a long i (as in c<u>y</u>clone), a long e (as in sill<u>y</u>), or as its own unique sound (as in yellow).	

TABLE 12.5   Sample Phonetic Teaching Materials

Elementary school
    Helping Children Overcome Learning Difficulties (Rosner)
    Word Express (Stemach and Williams)
Middle school
    Phonic Remedial Reading Lessons (Kirk et al.)
    Phonics Pathways (Hiskes)
    Phono Cards (Montgomery)
Adult education
    Sounds Like Word Books (Fidell)

Source: Academic Therapy Publishers, Novato, CA.

Additionally, reading level and spelling performance are assessed before instruction begins.

Classroom lessons are based on the level of the group being taught. All lessons involve the use of flashcards to familiarize students with the symbols, sounds, and rules of decoding. There are three phases to each 1-hour session. First, the children review the cards with printed symbols that they have not yet mastered. The instructor flashes cards to one child at a time in a round-robin fashion until the group can successfully identify the sounds associated with the letter on each card. Ten to 15 minutes are spent in this visual-auditory phase of instruction. Another method often used during this phase is called *decoding detec-*

Consonants

b__ c__ d__ f__ g__ h__ j__ k__ l__ m__ n__
p__ qu__ r__ s__ t__ v__ w__ x__ y__ z__

Vowels

a__ e__ i__ o__ u__

Consonant Blends and Digraphs

sh__ wh__ ch__ th__ st__ sl__ sp__ sw__ sm__ sn__ sc__
sk__ tr__ cr__ dr__ fr__ pr__ br__ gr__ fl__ gl__ pl__

cl__ bl__ tw__ spr__ thr__ scr__ str__ squ__ spl__ shr__

Final Consonant Sounds

ng__ nk__ mp__ nch__ ed__ nd__ nt__ pt__ ly__ ft__ sp__

st__ lt__ lk__ ct__ sk__ que__

Silent Consonant Sounds

kn__ gn__ wr__ mb__ tch__ ck__ igh__ bt__ rh__ mn__ stle_

Vowels Digraphs and Dipthongs

ee__ ai__ ea__ ay__ oa__ oo__ oy__ oe__ au__ oi__ ow__

ew__ ou__ ie__ aw__ ue__ ey__ ei__ vi__ eu__ gue__ qua__

R-Controlled Vowels

ar__ er__ ir__ er__ ur__ ear__ wor__ war__

Phonetic Irregularities

gh__ dge__ ph__ igh__ tion__ alk__ all__ ble__ ind__ sion__
eigh__ ough__ augh__

FIGURE 12.2
Modified instructional skills checklist.

tives: The teacher produces a sound and the student must pick the flashcard that corresponds to that sound. In the second phase, the auditory-tactile phase, letter or letter combination sounds are dictated for the child to write, which provides the multisensory combination of vision, hearing, movement, and touch to reinforce the symbol-sound relationship. This process is more involved than the traditional method of assuming the child will learn the word merely through persistent sight presentations. Ten to 15 minutes of the hour are devoted to the second phase. In the third phase, the student learns to spell words that involve the sounds, using rules from the first two phases of instruction. This phase requires approximately 15 minutes and is followed by the final activity of reading text. The teacher selects appropriate text for the students to read aloud, one at a time. The teacher fosters an environment in which the students all help each other and benefit from the suggestions of their peers as well as from suggestions of their own.

Using this methodology, the students work through all the levels and rules of English and learn the structure and logic of the written language. Confidence is fostered, and students are made to feel that, if they don't know how to spell a word, they can usually figure it out.

Efficacy of Multisensory Language Therapy

To our knowledge, the only study of the effects of multisensory language therapy on dyslexia (determined by a method of direct diagnosis) took place at the New Visions School. Fourteen students at the school were found to be among the most debilitated in terms of reading and spelling based on psychoeducational evaluations done before entering the school. The children ranged in grade placement from third to seventh (11 were in fifth through seventh grades). The DDT was used to determine the cause or causes of their RD, and all were found to have dysphoneidesia. Decoding levels ranged from primer to fifth grade, with the average being third grade. Pretreatment testing was also administered using the standard tests to determine percentile levels for reading and spelling. Throughout the entire school year (36 weeks), all 14 students were seen in groups of three or four for 1 hour of instruction with an education specialist. Post-testing with the DDT revealed an increase in decoding level of 1.96 years, as opposed to an average of 0.61 years of progress in each year before the multisensory intervention. This difference was statistically significant at the $p = 0.001$ level. Reading and spelling performance showed average gains of 16.6% and 27.6%, respectively. The improvements were impressive, but analysis of DDT patterns revealed that none of the 14 students were "cured" of their dyslexia. Dyslexic decoding and encoding patterns persisted. This finding lends credence to the notion that dyslexia is an entity that must be dealt with using a special approach. Of the 14 subjects, 12 remained dysphoneidetic on post-testing, one became only dyseidetic, and another only dysphonetic. It is not surprising for a dysphoneidetic dyslexic to have only a dyseidetic pattern after extensive therapy because dysphonesia is less genetic and more environmental in nature than dyseidesia. The finding of dysphonesia in the other case is less easily explained, but it is notable that the student's history revealed the presence of mild cerebral palsy and so this is atypical of cases of dyslexia.

The results of this study of multisensory language therapy for dyslexia demonstrate its capacity to help individuals ameliorate their RD. Nonetheless, the language therapy is not to be viewed as a cure for dyslexia. A combination of intersensory integrative therapy (e.g., optometric vision therapy and occupational therapy) with multisensory language therapy often provides the best opportunity for individuals to achieve an acceptable measure of mastery of the written language. Some of the following case studies exemplify the hopeful prospect that dyslexic individuals can lead productive and rewarding lives.

Case Studies

Each of the five patients in the sample cases in this section were seen by at least one of the authors. Only highlights and pertinent information are presented to clarify and emphasize the principal points of optometric management for each case.

Case 1: Nondyslexia with Reading Dysfunction

Erica, 13 years old and in the eighth grade, presented with complaints of eye fatigue while performing near work. Further questioning elicited the observation from her mother that Erica had great difficulty with reading, math, and completing assignments in school. Erica was receiving 1 hour per day of special educational service for poor reading and course work at school. She had migraine headaches and took medication to improve her complexion.

Optometric evaluation showed compound myopic astigmatism of the right eye and simple myopia of the left eye, convergence excess, saccadic and VPM problems, and no indication of dyslexia, on TDS.[4]

In a consultation with Erica's parents, the diagnosis and prognosis were explained and a plan of therapy devised. Treatment included vision therapy to address problems in binocularity, saccades, visual memory, visual-motor integration, and auditory-visual integration. Some time was planned to help Erica develop and use memory skills, specifically for test taking, as well as strategies for reading to learn (such as surveying the material first, questioning while reading, and reviewing material when needed). The estimated treatment time was 32 office visits with prescribed therapy every day at home.

Results of 32 visits of vision therapy are represented in Tables 12.6 and 12.7. These data show that most VSE and VPM functions were improved; saccades were somewhat less improved. Erica's reading and comprehension and her overall school grades improved.

Case 2: Dyseidesia

Bob was initially seen for an evaluation related to his difficulty with school work. At the time of this evaluation he was 10 years old and in the fifth grade. His academic history was significant in that he had received special reading services throughout his school career. Medical history was noncontributory, and he had a normal birth history. Bob's older brother had confirmed dyseidesia with formal testing on the DDT. The father was also strongly suspected of having dyslexia, although formal testing was never performed.

Bob's symptoms included eye rubbing, avoidance of near work, eyestrain after near work, losing his place while reading, and spelling and reading problems. Pertinent clinical findings are displayed in

TABLE 12.6   Vision Skills Efficiency Findings, Case 1

Pertinent Pretherapy Findings			Post-Therapy
Symptoms			
Eye fatigue associated with near work			Completely eliminated
Difficulty staying on task			Much better
Working too slowly and with excessive effort			Much better
Visual acuity, habitual	6 m	40 cm	
OD −0.75 − 0.50 × 100	20/25	20/20	
OS −1.00 − 0.50 × 167	20/25	20/20	
NPC (break/recovery)			
3 cm with diplopia			To nose
Refraction			
OD −1.25 − 1.00 × 100	20/20		Same
OS −1.75 DS	20/20		Same
Phorometry			
6 m 1 esophoria, no hyper			Orthophoria
40 cm 2 esophoria, no hyper			Same
BI vergence 12/21/0			16/20/12
BO vergence 26/28/16			16/25/20
NRA +3.00			+3.00
PRA −1.50			−2.00
Accommodative facility (±2.00)			
OD 6 cpm			8.5 cpm
OS 6 cpm			10 cpm
Developmental Eye Movement Test			
A = 21 secs			A = 18 secs
B = 27 secs			B = 18 secs
C = 59 secs			C = 42 secs (also significant improvement in visual-verbal automaticity reflected in lower A, B, and C times)
ratio = 1.23			ratio = 1.17
10th percentile			20th percentile

NPC = near point convergence; BI = base-in; BO = base-out; NRA = negative relative accommodation; PRA = positive relative accommodation; cpm = cycles per minute.

Tables 12.8 and 12.9. The initial findings support the diagnoses of (1) simple hyperopia, (2) convergence insufficiency, (3) accommodative infacility, (4) poor saccadic eye movements, and (5) VPM problems. Dyslexia testing using form A of the DDT revealed moderate dyseidesia (Table 12.10).

A plan of treatment was devised and discussed with the parents. A spectacle prescription was written for use while in the classroom and for near work outside the classroom (OD +0.50, OS +0.75). Vision therapy to address the VSE and VPM problems was estimated to require

TABLE 12.7 Visual-Perceptual-Motor Findings Before and After Therapy, Case 1

Pertinent Pretherapy Findings	Post-Therapy	Change
Reversal Frequency Test (Gardner)		
Recognition 14th percentile	78th percentile	+64 percentile points
Visual sequential memory (TVAS)		
50th percentile	75th percentile	+25 percentile points
Getman Visualization test		
Age equivalent 7	12	+5 yrs
Visual-motor integration (Beery)		
4th percentile	70th percentile	+66 percentile points
Auditory-visual integration (Birch-Belmont)		
20th percentile	80th percentile	+60 percentile points
Visual concentration (Groffman)		
Age equivalent 10	13	+3 yrs

TVAS = Test of Visual Analysis Skills.

TABLE 12.8 Visual Skills Efficiency Findings Before and After Therapy, Case 2

Pertinent Pretherapy Findings	Post-Therapy
Symptoms	
Rubs eyes, eyestrain after near work, loses place, avoids near work, poor reading and spelling	All visual symptoms eliminated; reading and spelling improved
Visual acuity	
6 m 20/20 OD, OS, binocular	Same
40 cm 20/20 OD, OS, binocular	Same
NPC 3 cm with diplopia	To nose
Refraction	
Ret OD +0.75 OS +1.00	
Subjective OD +0.50 20/20	Same
OS +0.75 20/20	
Phorometry	
6 m orthophoria, no hyperphoria	Same
40 cm 8$^\Delta$ exophoria	3$^\Delta$ exophoria
BO vergence 15/20/–3	x/19/13
BI vergence x/16/15	x/20/6
NRA +2.00	+2.00 D
PRA –1.75	–2.00 D
Accommodative facility	
OD 7 cpm	11 cpm
OS 5 cpm (more difficulty with plus)	10.5 cpm
Developmental eye movement test	
A = 21	A = 19
B = 27	B = 21
C = 59	C = 44
Ratio = 1.23	Ratio = 1.10
30th percentile	55th percentile

NPC = near point convergence; BI = base-in; BO = base-out; NRA = negative relative accommodation; PRA = positive relative accommodation; cpm = cycles per minute.

TABLE 12.9 Visual-Perceptual-Motor Findings Before and After Therapy, Case 2

Pretherapy	Post-Therapy	Change
Reversal Frequency Test		
Recognition 25th percentile	72nd percentile	+47 percentile points
Visual sequential memory		
25th percentile	63rd percentile	+38 percentile points
Getman Visualization Test		
Age equivalent 7	12	+5 yrs
Visual-motor integration		
6th percentile	19th percentile	+13 percentile points
Auditory-visual integration		
20th percentile	70th percentile	+50 percentile points
Visual concentration (Groffman tracings)		
Age equivalent 12	13	+1 yr

TABLE 12.10 Pretherapy and Post-Therapy Dyslexia Findings, Case 2

Pretherapy	Post-Therapy (7 months later)
Decoding	
Third grade	Fifth grade
Encoding	
Eidetic 20%	0%
Phonetic 80%	70%
Diagnosis	
Moderate dyseidesia	Moderate dyseidesia

32–36 visits. The patient and parents were informed of the apparent dyslexic pattern and told not to expect a cure of the dyslexia as a result of vision therapy. The therapy was designed to eliminate the contributory vision problems and to serve as a foundation for multisensory, phonetic language therapy in school to address the problem of dyslexia.

Results of the 32 office visits of vision therapy indicate successful management of most of the contributory visual problems in Bob's case. Although subjective visual symptoms were largely eliminated, the spelling and reading problems persisted. The pattern of dyseidesia remained unchanged, as expected (Table 12.10). The parents were not dissatisfied with the results because they had been counseled about expectations before vision therapy began. They received a post-therapy progress letter and addendum with suggestions for educational therapy to address the dyslexia, which opened a helpful dialogue with the school system.

This case demonstrates the successful programming of vision therapy to eliminate contributory vision problems in the case of dyseidesia. It also underscores the importance of follow-up educational services to address the written language problems that result from dyslexia.

Successful educational programming for the child with dyslexia depends on resources of the local school district, the vigilance of the parents, the concern of outside professionals, and the level of cooperation attainable with the professionals in decision-making positions in the school.

Case 3: Dysphoneidesia

Donald was first seen for dyslexia testing and a VPM evaluation when he was 8.5 years old. He was in the third grade at the time and had a long history of reading problems in school. The DDT results showed a mild dyseidetic pattern along with a mild dysphonetic pattern. Donald was unable to complete the alphabet, either orally or in writing. The letters he did know were written correctly with no reversals, but there were six omissions of uppercase letters and seven omissions of lowercase letters. Donald had some vision problems, mainly in the area of poor accommodative facility. The Piaget right-left awareness test showed some poor laterality and directionality. The Beery Developmental Visual-Motor Integration Test also indicated problems.

Donald's parents were advised that accommodative facility therapy was recommended and that further testing by a multidisciplinary team should be performed. The team was to consider therapy for visual-motor integration, laterality, directionality, and special educational therapy for dyseidesia and dysphonesia.

Testing by a school psychologist revealed that Donald had above-average intelligence; the verbal scale on the Wechsler Intelligence Scale for Children–Revised was 113 and the performance scale was 115. Donald had a composite percentile rank of 70 on the Iowa Tests of Basic Skills.

Donald's parents enrolled him in a special private school for additional education and tutoring in addition to public school. The educational therapy emphasized computer-assisted instruction in reading and language arts. During the next few years, his parents also enrolled him in several other programs. One of these was the Structure of the Intellect (SOI) Institute. Testing revealed weak areas that included visual closure, visual discrimination, visual concentration for sequencing, symbol pattern discrimination, auditory sequencing, judgment of arithmetic similarities, and form reasoning. Subsequent to the SOI evaluation, Donald had a thorough neurologic workup in the pediatric department of a local general hospital. The neurologist reported a finding of dysgraphia, with other areas normal, and a diagnosis of delayed neurologic maturation with a central processing deficit. The advice given was to continue with the private educational tutoring.

Because our clinic was far from his home, Donald and his parents elected to have vision therapy provided by a nearby optometric specialist. The vision therapy continued for several months and addressed the accommodative, laterality, directionality, and visual-motor integration problems. Donald's local optometrist saw him periodically for the next 6 years.

When Donald was 14 years old, he returned to our clinic for retesting with the DDT. By then, he was in the ninth grade, enrolled full time in a private school that provided intensive personalized instruction, with about 2 hours per week of additional tutoring in reading. He said he still had trouble reading, writing, and spelling and he described himself as a slow reader and poor speller. DDT results indicated that Donald was recognizing words at his grade placement for both eidetic and phonetic decoding, which was very encouraging. On encoding, however, a definite dyseidetic pattern was revealed (as was shown when he was in the third grade). He had 20% accuracy (mild severity) on the dictated eidetic words and 70% accuracy (normal considering the decoding level) on dictated phonetic words. Furthermore, he still had trouble writing the alphabet completely (one omission). The mild dyseidetic pattern remained unchanged, but the previous dysphonetic pattern appeared to have been eliminated. The efforts of educational therapy in the past, with emphasis on phonetic training, undoubtedly helped Donald to achieve an adequate level of phonetic performance. Donald apparently was able to achieve in school by means of diligent study habits and special help, including optometric intervention and continued tutoring in reading. He seemed to be very motivated to do well in school.

It is sometimes possible to modify dysphonesia through environmental intervention. There is less genetic influence in this pattern than in dyseidesia. It is reasonable to assume that the mild dysphonetic pattern found 6 years before had been eliminated as a result of the extensive special training Donald received. Dyseidesia, on the other hand, rarely goes away, either with time or as the result of training (any kind of therapy). This dyslexic pattern seems to be transmitted genetically in the autosomal dominant mode. Theoretically, 50% of the children of an affected parent will show an autosomal dominant trait, such as dyseidesia. Donald's father was tested with the ADT and found to have a similar dyseidetic pattern. His encoding results showed 30% eidetic accuracy and 70% phonetic accuracy.

Donald has been able to improve his phonetic abilities, but his eidetic problems in reading, writing, and spelling remain. Fortunately, he has only a mild dyseidetic dyslexia, which is not severely handicapping. Nevertheless, Donald has trouble matching whole-word visual gestalts with whole-word auditory gestalts (which is the definition of dyseidesia). Because the dyseidesia is mild, Donald is able to decode and encode many words eidetically. Unknown words must be decoded and encoded phonetically, and he often depends on the support of motoric memory by writing cursively to spell words correctly. This tactile-kinesthetic support is important for him to achieve in reading, writing, and spelling.

Suggestions given were to continue using cursive writing for his motoric memory flow and to take full advantage of tactual and kinesthetic input and output. The use of a computer to check spelling errors and the use of a tape recorder to assist in note taking were advised. Donald had no trouble listening and understanding what was said to him, but reading printed material and writing with correct spelling remained a problem. Donald was advised to continue with a tutor well versed in phonics. It was hoped that Donald could master all the phonetic rules of the English language. When phonetic rules are applied, approximately 80% of the words in the English language (at one's grade placement) can be spelled correctly. This is normal performance, even for nondyslexic individuals. Donald should be able to decode many unfamiliar words by knowing and applying phonetic rules. Donald's strength areas in reading and spelling were his phonetic and motoric abilities. His weak area was in the eidetic ability for word recognition (decoding) and revisualizing the orthography of words for spelling (encoding).

Educational therapy should emphasize the strengths of phonetic and motoric skills. When these are mastered, an eidetic approach may then be emphasized. The use of flash cards would help Donald develop a larger sight vocabulary. Tedious drills would be necessary for Donald to learn new words, but he could become frustrated when the eidetic approach alone is used to improve his reading vocabulary. He needs to resort to his phonetic and motoric strengths as backup.

These suggestions were made to his teachers and parents: Donald should continue learning to work around his dyseidetic problem as he has been doing, but the team (composed of parents, teachers, concerned health professionals, and Donald himself) must realize that Donald's reading will necessarily be slower than normal (by approximately one-third of the normally expected time) and that spelling will probably continue to be a problem for him. If he is given extra time to complete a lengthy written test, such as a long multiple-choice exam, Donald should be able to achieve high scores. His intellectual abilities allow good comprehension once the written words are decoded. There is every reason for Donald to succeed academically if the nature of his dyseidesia is understood and worked around with the help of appropriate educational therapy and the use of supports such as tape recorders, computers, and study groups.

Donald returned again for dyslexia testing at the age of 19.5 years. At that time he was beginning his second year of college. The ADT was given, and Donald was found to be decoding at high school level. On the encoding portion, Donald did well on the phonetic results, but a dyseidetic pattern continued to be evident.

To determine whether there was any problem with visual memory or visual-motor integration, the Monroe Visual III Test (see Appendix) was administered, and Donald did very well: he drew 15 of the 16 nonlinguistic figures correctly. He is probably better than average on this type of visual memory. Donald's visual memory for language symbols (words) remains a problem, however. Donald still reports having some difficulty in school, although he is a hard-working student. He did well in his business courses in a small private college in his first year. His grades were fairly good, although English was his most difficult course. He is still a relatively slow reader and uses the dictionary a great deal to check his spelling. He comprehends well once things are told to him and is getting fairly good grades.

At the time of the college-age visit, Donald had recently seen an ophthalmologist, who prescribed reading glasses. He did not bring them in, so the spectacle lens prescription was not known. These lenses were apparently prescribed to relieve headaches but, according to Donald, they were not much help and he did not wear his eyeglasses regularly. Although he did have some complaints of headaches at one time, he has no ocular problems now and feels that he does not need to wear spectacles. A refraction was done and the results were

OD	−0.25	−0.25 × 90	20/20+
OS	−0.25	−0.25 × 90	20/20

His unaided visual acuity was 20/20⁻ in each eye. There was a slight degree of myopic astigmatism but probably not enough to warrant wearing glasses. A family history of myopia may mean that Donald will develop more myopia later in his college career. Donald was advised to be aware of his distant visual acuity compared with that of his peers and, if he has a noticeable problem seeing things far away (particularly road signs at night), a spectacle lens correction may then be advised for certain tasks at far distances. A small degree of myopia, however, should have little or no adverse affect on his near work, such as reading. It does not appear that Donald needs reading lenses at this time for his near work tasks.

Back in the third grade, laterality and directionality problems were evident. Retesting on the Piaget right-left awareness test showed that Donald now has no difficulty in this area. He claims that study of anatomy and learning to visualize the structure of the heart helped him to learn directionality of symbols and eliminated his right and left confusion.

Donald was asked to write the alphabet. He slowly wrote the small lowercase letters from a to z neatly and with no reversals, but he omitted v and x. Donald was advised to learn to say the alphabet orally and learn to write and practice it until the alphabet becomes automatic to him. This skill is important for looking up words in the dictionary or alphabetizing written material.

Because Donald is doing relatively well in school at this time, further educational therapy is probably unnecessary, but helpful hints for someone who has a dyseidetic pattern follow. In Donald's studies, he should use every means possible to work around the handicapping condition of dyseidesia. He should have people study with him and read aloud to him and have others talk with him about the subject matter. He should use tape recorders as much as possible and use all means available to get the meaning of the written message. Even though it may take a little longer at times, it is important for Donald to repeat his reading tasks until he grasps the meaning of his assignments. It may be that very lengthy tests, such as multiple-choice tests, take longer for him to complete. Donald should talk to his teachers in advance and request that testing times be modified when a large amount of reading is required.

Donald is doing well in school, but he has to be aware of his mild eidetic coding problems and how they slow his reading and interfere with consistently good spelling.

Follow-up reports show that Donald finished college with a bachelor's degree in business. He is now employed and doing well in his occupation and his personal life.

Case 4: Dysnemkinphoneidesia

June was 8 years old and in the second grade when she was referred because of reduced visual acuity. No other visual symptoms were reported. She had been previously diagnosed with dyslexia and was receiving special reading instruction at school in half-hour sessions three times per week. June had repeated the first grade because of reading difficulties, but math and other subjects were not a problem. June's personal eye history was unremarkable except for a spectacle correction to be used for reading, which was prescribed when she was 6 years old. She discontinued the use of her glasses for unspecified reasons. Her medical history revealed frequent ear infections from birth to 18 months of age. She had anemia when she was 3 and 4 years old, and had a current prescription for diphenhydramine (Benadryl) to "help her stay on task." No pertinent family eye or health history was elicited.

The initial vision examination revealed unaided visual acuities of 20/25 at far and 20/20 at near in each eye. The subjective refraction yielded:

OD	+2.00 –0.75 × 095	20/15
OS	+1.75 –0.75 × 090	20/15

June also exhibited deficient saccades (undershooting), pursuits (unsteady), reduced positive relative accommodation (PRA) (–1.00 D), and positive and negative fusional vergences as follows:

	6 m	40 cm
Base-in	x/4/2	8/14/6
Base-out	6/12/3	16/22/10

The subjective refraction resulted in a prescription that was cut by a half diopter in the sphere power and a quarter diopter in the cylinder power; this was prescribed mainly for reading. June was also referred for a VSE evaluation, VPM evaluation, and testing with the DDT.

Supplemental history from June's parents and teachers indicated problems in reading, with an estimated level of mid–first grade. Additional visual symptoms included loss of place when reading, use of a finger to keep place, rereading and skipping lines, discomfort with visual tasks, holding reading material too close, copying errors, short attention span, and poor handwriting.

The VSE evaluation revealed deficiencies in pursuit and saccadic eye movement skills, accommodative infacility, poor PRA, and poor negative fusional vergence. The VPM evaluation revealed weakness in laterality, directionality, letter reversals, visual-motor integration, visual-motor speed and precision, and gross motor skills and difficulty with sentence copy tasks. Dyslexia testing revealed a decoding level of first grade (relatively equal eidetic and phonetic decoding modes) with below age-expected performance on the nemkinesia testing due to abnormally high number and letter reversals. Encoding results suggested mild deficits in eidetic and phonetic processes. A diagnosis of dysnemkinphoneidesia was made. A vision therapy program consisting of one 45-minute session per week was recommended to improve the deficient VSE and VPM skills and dysnemkinesia. Recommendations for educational therapy were also made to address the dyslexic components of dysphonesia and dyseidesia.

June had 20 vision therapy sessions during the next 6 months. The following vision therapy activities (some not discussed in this text) were performed in office and home vision training.

Pursuits   Pencil pursuits, pie pan rotations, marble roll, pegboard rotator, and Marsden ball pursuits
Saccades   Pencil saccades, corner saccades, Hart chart saccades, La Barge Electrotherapist, Michigan tracking, and continuous motion line drawing
Accommodation   Robbins phoropter rock and accommodative flipper rock
Vergence   Vectograms, Wheatstone stereoscope, Tranaglyphs, Remy separator, and Eccentric Circle fusion activities
Gross motor and bilateral integration   Balance beam and balance board activities, marching patterns, ball bounce, snow angels, and jumping jacks
Laterality/Directionality   Floor map, Simon says, Kirschner arrows, La Barge Electrotherapist, Landolt C's, Money road map, and letter finds
Visual-motor integration   Perceptuomotor Pen tracing, continuous motion line drawing, haptic writing, and Rosner program

The first progress evaluation after 5 weeks of vision therapy showed that deficiencies in pursuit abilities were eliminated; saccades, laterality, and directionality of letters were improved. No change was evident in gross motor and accommodative skills.

The second progress evaluation after five more vision therapy sessions indicated that saccadic, laterality, directionality, and letter reversal deficits were eliminated. Improvements were also made in accommodative skills. The DDT was administered again. The decoding level had improved to second grade, and there was no evidence of dysnemkinesia. The pattern of dysphoneidesia, however, persisted; severity remained mild.

The third progress evaluation after another five vision therapy sessions revealed that deficits in accommodation, negative fusional vergence, and gross motor skills were eliminated. There were also improvements in visual-motor integration.

A progress evaluation was performed 1 year later. All previous visual symptoms were reported to be eliminated and reading skills were reportedly better. June was still involved in an educational therapy program at school to address her specific RD. Testing revealed some regression in pursuits, saccades, directionality, and letter reversals from the improvements made in vision therapy. Only accommodative skills remained completely normal. It was recommended that June resume a vision therapy program to remedy these vision problems. For unknown reasons, these recommendations were not followed.

June was seen 6 years later for a primary care vision examination. She presented with complaints of blur at far. Unfortunately, there was no follow-up on the previous visual symptoms or reading difficulties, but a new lens prescription was written for use in school:

OD   Plano −0.50 × 090   20/20
OS   +0.50 −1.25 × 090   20/20

June was contacted 7 years later and advised to have a follow-up evaluation of her dyslexia. She was 21 years old and reported that she still had difficulties with reading, writing, and spelling but no trouble with letter reversals. She uses an audiotape service from the Braille Institute and takes only one class at a time at her community junior college, where she has completed 18 of the 30 units necessary for a nursery school instructor's certificate. She has had intelligence testing performed at a local university counseling service and was found to have normal intelligence. She reported that she is still easily distracted when reading, but background music helps her concentration. The ADT revealed a fourth-grade decoding level. Encoding results of the ADT showed a marked pattern of dyseidesia and a mild-to-moderate pattern of dysphonesia.

It can be concluded from this case that optometric vision therapy helps to lessen the contributing problems of RD and that a dyslexic individual—even one with dysnemkinphoneidesia, the most severe type of dyslexia—can achieve success with appropriate therapies, both optometric and educational.

Case 5: Adult with Dyslexia and Tinted Lenses

This case report revolves around the discussion of tinted lenses in dyslexia. Laura is a 28-year-old dyseidetic female who uses tinted lenses from the Irlen Institute for "dyslexia." Before discussing Laura's case, background information on tinted lenses is presented.

Meares[31] claimed that many children with dyslexia were able to improve their reading by placing frosted plastic sheets (to reduce visibility by lowering the contrast between the print and the page) over their reading materials (refer to discussions on magnocellular deficits in Chapters 4 and 5). Irlen[32] claimed that tinted lenses were effective in treating a condition she called the *scotopic sensitivity syndrome* (SSS). She maintains that SSS is composed of a number of visual-perceptual disturbances prevalent among individuals with dyslexia. Since 1983, tinted lenses have been used in Australia to treat individuals with "dyslexia."[33] This treatment caught on in the United States, largely aided by a *60 Minutes* television broadcast in 1988, which publicized *anecdotal* successes of the Irlen lens regimen.

Our purpose here is to clarify the confusion surrounding this method of treatment. We provide information that will allow professionals, parents of dyslexic children, and persons with dyslexia to judge the claims made by businesses that market and distribute tinted lenses.

Scientific Basis of Scotopic Sensitivity Syndrome

Rosner and Rosner[34] provided a review of the literature on the Irlen tinted-lens treatment. They concluded, "We would join countless others in applauding a discovery which helped solve the riddle these LD children present. But, we have also seen a number of miracle 'cures' (panaceas) burst upon the scene, be heralded (typically by the developers and marketers of the cure), and then fade away. We have no reason to condemn the Irlen treatment; but neither do we have any reason to recommend it." The Rosners expressed concern regarding Irlen's lack of definition of the symptoms used in the diagnosis of SSS (i.e., poor visual resolution, depth perception, sustained focus, span of focus, peripheral vision, and eyestrain), her failure to explain the composition of her diagnostic battery (the Irlen Differential Perceptual Schedule) for determining the appropriate therapeutic lens tint, and her failure to describe how the subjects were checked for improvement in their symptoms after application of the tinted lenses. Rosner and Rosner also indicated that the unscientific approach used effectively precluded a replication study. Furthermore, claims of improvement due to treatment were based solely on subjective reports of the clients rather than on quantitative statistics from objective tests. This calls the validity of Irlen's findings into question.

Fitzgerald[33] reviewed tinted lenses and dyslexia. She discussed studies that showed some improvements in reading functions as a result of tinted-lens treatment.[31, 32, 35-39] Closer inspection of one study showed that word matching and letter recognition improved, but word recognition was unchanged.[36] In another, Stanley[38] found that "quite real motivational effects are produced when colored filters are used, but the basic problems of reading disability are not removed." Cheetham and Ovenden[37] agreed that although the tinted lenses could help facilitate reading in poor readers, they did not cure the reading problem.

Wilsher and Taylor,[40] however, demonstrated no improvement in reading ability. Another study by a group known as SPELD[41] showed no statistically significant difference in reading rate, comprehension, or accuracy between their experimental tinted-lens group and a control group. Reading assessment was performed using the Neale Analysis of Reading after one and two school terms (total 6 months). This study also found that only 11 of the 24 subjects continued to wear prescribed tinted lenses by the end of the second term.

Although these controlled studies appear to negate reports of improvement in reading function due to tinted lenses, it does appear that certain individuals may experience some improvement as a result of wearing the lenses.[41] Cardinal et al.[42] addressed the possible explanations for these improvements. Three possibilities are (1) the tinted lenses filter out the specific wavelengths to which the person with SSS is sensitive, (2) the tinted lenses improve visual functions related to the symptoms that Irlen attributes to SSS, or (3) the placebo effect.

Tinted lenses filter only some of the light at a particular wavelength.[43] Even with very dark tints (e.g., 75% of white light filtered out), some light of all wavelengths passes through the lens. Therefore the theory that the lenses work by filtering *out* a band of light is questionable. Furthermore the notion of a condition, SSS, causing visual disturbances while reading does not make sense from a logical standpoint. *Scotopic* refers to a physiologic characteristic of "scotopic vision, or the levels of illumination at which the eye is dark adapted."[44] Dark adaptation gradually occurs over a period of 30–40 minutes when an individual is removed from a normally illuminated environment and is placed in a dark one. The retinal receptors required for reading are the cones, which provide distinct central vision in normal lighting. They are deactivated in the dark, which allows the peripherally located retinal receptors (the rods) to become activated. The rods provide visual processing under low illumination or night vision conditions. Reading does not normally occur under conditions of dark adaptation. Hence, the semantic basis for SSS is questionable.

Visual Dysfunctions and Scotopic Sensitivity Syndrome

Evidence contradicts the assertion that tinted lenses improve vision functions. Scheiman et al.[45] demonstrated in their study of 37 subjects who tested positive for SSS that 95% were found to have some or all of the following: significant refractive errors (need for corrective spectacle lenses), accommodative (eye focusing) dysfunctions, and binocular (eye-teaming) anomalies. They pointed out that Irlen's SSS symptom list (e.g., headaches, words doubling, words blurring, words moving, and tiring while reading) is nearly identical to disturbances experienced by individuals with the above-mentioned refractive, accommodative, and binocular problems.[45] Furthermore, Blaskey et al.[46] investigated the efficacy of vision therapy in lieu of Irlen lenses for treating SSS. Subjects who tested positive for SSS were randomly assigned either to a vision therapy program or a control group. Measurements of visual functions, symptoms, reading performance on standardized tests, and SSS indices were made before and after treatment. Based on these findings of visual function, it appears that Irlen may have redefined VSE problems as SSS. It is important to note that, in a report of 238 references, vision therapy was shown to be valid and efficacious in the treatment of VSE anomalies.[47]

Effectiveness of Tinted Lenses

We believe that the placebo effect is at work in the tinted-lens treatment. Psychological factors are involved: Wearing the lenses allows the individual with dyslexia to eliminate the stigma of a hidden handicap by making the problem obvious so that the individual is more likely to be treated with compassion. Stanley[38] indicated that many of the subjects wanted the lenses to work and therefore were increasingly motivated to work and study hard. Fitzgerald[33] reported that many tinted-lens wearers showed great increases in self-esteem, perhaps due to increased concern by others for the problem or the hope of being cured, despite no improvement in reading.

From our experience, the Irlen lens treatment does not appear to cure dyslexia. This conclusion comes as no surprise in light of the strong evidence indicating a neuroanatomic basis for dyslexia. Fitzgerald[43] indicated that, based on neuroanatomic evidence, there may never be a cure for dyslexia. Nevertheless, early diagnosis to prevent secondary emotional problems is essential.[17] Multidisciplinary care can then allow for development of full learning potential.

Despite the evidence contrary to the Irlen lens treatment as a cure for dyslexia, further investigation for possible benefits from this treatment should be carried out. Gole et al.[41] found a subgroup of poor readers (among 1,200 children studied) who benefited from the use of the tinted lenses. This notion might explain the confused reporting indicated by various studies that fail to agree on the effects of the Irlen lenses. The problem of lumping together various types of poor readers has plagued research in this area.[48] If there is one type of poor reader who may be improved by the Irlen lens treatment, then efforts should be made to identify types of RD as a part of the research design.

Eidetic Encoding   Phonetic Encoding

1. _prerequisite_   c   1. _lutigeous_   e

2. _mannechin (manneguin)_   2. _tinkchur_   c

3. _nostic (gnostic)_   3. _ollagarkey_   c

4. _parlement (parliament)_   4. _eneffacashus_   c

5. _endeavor_   c   5. _parchurishun_   c

6. _regime_   c   6. _homeopothee_   c

7. _exonerate_   c   7. _evaness_   c

     _57_ % correct   _100_ % correct

Refer to Table 7. (Interpretation of Encoding Scores for Classification of Severity of Dyslexia) to relate encoding % correct with decoding level.

Eidetic Coding	Phonetic Coding
☐ Above Normal	☑ Above Normal
☐ Normal	☐ Normal
☐ Borderline-Normal	☐ Borderline-Normal
☑ Mild Severity	☐ Mild Severity
☐ Mild-Moderate Severity	☐ Mild-Moderate Severity
☐ Moderate Severity	☐ Moderate Severity
☐ Moderate-Marked Severity	☐ Moderate-Marked Severity
☐ Marked Severity	☐ Marked Severity

Name of Examinee __Laura__   Age _28_ Date _4/27/90_

FIGURE 12.3
Encoding and interpretation results of testing with the Adult Dyslexia Test in a case of dyseidetic dyslexia.

Case Discussion

Laura had been an Irlen client. We were able to diagnose her dyslexia after her SSS evaluation and tinted-lens use for 2 years, using the ADT.[10] Comparisons of decoding ability with and without the tinted lenses were made as well as a comparison of coding patterns to those of a friend of Laura who is nondyslexic.

Laura graduated from college at age 25, earning a bachelor's degree in English. She works in the film industry as a script reviewer. As a child she had difficulty learning to read and spell, although math was never a problem, and was only able to pursue her education and career through great perseverance. She reported that she had speech and language therapy in grade school and remembers failing many tests. Her father has similar difficulty in reading and spelling (possible genetic dyslexic trait).

Results of the ADT (Figure 12.3) for Laura revealed a mild dyseidesia. In this type of dyslexia, the individual has difficulty matching

Eidetic Encoding   Phonetic Encoding

1. __mimicry__ c   1. __homiopothy__ c
2. __demagogue__ c   2. __evaness__ c
3. __oligarchy__ c   3. __geodicy__ c
4. __tincture__ c   4. __coolum__ c
5. __litigious__ c   5. __exte exactabel__ c
6. __rhapsody__ c   6. __delaguess__ c
7. __prerequisite__ c   7. __calleguy__ c

__100__ % correct   __100__ % correct

Refer to Table 7. (Interpretation of Encoding Scores for Classification of Severity of Dyslexia) to relate encoding % correct with decoding level.

Eidetic Coding	Phonetic Coding
☑ Above Normal	☑ Above Normal
☐ Normal	☐ Normal
☐ Borderline-Normal	☐ Borderline-Normal
☐ Mild Severity	☐ Mild Severity
☐ Mild-Moderate Severity	☐ Mild-Moderate Severity
☐ Moderate Severity	☐ Moderate Severity
☐ Moderate-Marked Severity	☐ Moderate-Marked Severity
☐ Marked Severity	☐ Marked Severity

Name of Examinee __Alice__   Age __25__ Date __4/27/90__

FIGURE 12.4
Encoding and inter-pretation results of testing with the Adult Dyslexia Test in a case with no indica-tion of dyslexia.

whole-word auditory gestalts, but the use of phonetic word attack (phonics, syllabication, structural analysis, and blending) is intact.

In comparison, Alice is a 25-year-old female, also with a bachelor's degree in English, who has the same occupation as Laura with approx-imately the same duration of script-reviewing experience. Alice has no history of any difficulty learning to read or spell. She graduated from college at age 22. Figure 12.4 shows her ADT results.

A comparison of coding in both cases reveals that Laura was decod-ing at lower-division college level and Alice was decoding at upper-division college level. Both were given an estimated grade placement of master's level based on their formal education (post-graduate cours-es) and extensive occupational experience. This grade placement esti-mation is made to determine if the individual is decoding at, above, or below the appropriate level. Diagnosis of the type and severity of dyslexia can be made by evaluating the eidetic and phonetic encoding patterns (see Figure 12.3) and using the ADT interpretation of encoding scores for classification of severity of dyslexia. Laura was decoding two levels below her estimated grade placement; this combined with her encoding scores of 57% eidetic and 100% phonetic indicates mild dyseidesia. Alice, on the other hand, was decoding only one level below her estimated grade placement, with encoding scores of 100% eidetic and 100% phonetic, indicating no dyslexia.

Laura repeated the decoding portion of the ADT while wearing her Irlen lenses; there was no difference in decoding ability (even though she had performed the same test about 1 hour before). She again decoded two levels below her expected grade placement. She was observed while reading text, with and without the Irlen lenses, and there was no appreciable difference in her speed or accuracy of decoding, but she did report that the tinted lenses seemed to make reading slightly more comfortable and "kept the words from floating." Laura was observed (casually and without her being placed in a testing situation) over several periods. She was never seen wearing the Irlen lenses for manuscript reading. She did use them as sunglasses when she went outdoors.

Further testing revealed that Laura had a mild convergence insufficiency. Alice also had a mild convergence insufficiency. Alice reported the same effect of slightly more comfort when reading through Laura's tinted lenses (a rust-blue color resembling sunglasses of medium darkness). Alice was advised to have vision therapy to eliminate her symptoms of eyestrain and blurred vision after reading; this was also recommended for Laura.

These case examples support our opinion that Irlen lenses do not cure dyslexia, although individuals who wear them often report some subjective improvement, which they attribute to the lenses. Additionally, reports of increased incidence of VSE problems among people diagnosed with SSS is supported. The use of the ADT in Laura's case provides a diagnosis supported by the educational and family history and allows for appropriate counseling, proper educational therapy, and implementation of compensatory measures.

Fortunately for Laura, her dyslexia is only mild, and she has already worked around it to a great extent. She explained that in college she did this by listening carefully in class and checking out required books to read before taking a particular class. Laura also used word processors with spell-checking programs to "survive" her composition and creative writing classes. English was her choice as a major because she felt she could apply contextual analysis to understand material in story form better than she could handle the technical reading in science courses. Furthermore, the pursuit of a career in television and film was not a major hardship, as Laura explained, because many of the books were the same as those she had in the lower division courses of her English major and much of television and film work was mechanical.

Another point exemplified in this case is that dyseidesia rarely, if ever, disappears from childhood to adulthood. The characteristic dyseidetic coding pattern remains. Nevertheless, in mild cases of dyslexia, individuals may be able, through great effort, to develop a sufficient sight-word lexicon to allow for reading of advanced materials. Even in more severe cases, it is possible that individuals with dyslexia may be able to pursue their chosen fields, when provided with the appropriate diagnosis and educational therapy.

Conclusions

Although opinion is mixed regarding the benefits of the Irlen lens treatment, the notion of the Irlen lens being a cure for dyslexia has no basis. Generally, the treatment does not significantly improve reading, even though some reports indicate improvement in a few reading-related tasks. Evidence indicating that the placebo effect is responsible for reading improvements cannot be dismissed. Efforts should be continued to determine whether or not there exists a subgroup of poor readers who are without symptoms related to visual dysfunctions and who are helped by the Irlen treatment for reasons other than the placebo effect.

Another area of concern is the fact that VSE anomalies have been shown to cause symptoms similar to those Irlen attributes to SSS. Symptoms such as headaches, blurred vision, eyestrain, and double vision are often associated with VSE problems and not necessarily with SSS. That Irlen may have simply redefined VSE anomalies as SSS is a distinct possibility.[46] Vision dysfunctions, such as vergence, accommodative, and ocular motor anomalies, may be remediated with optometric vision therapy. This is important for affected nondyslexic individuals and even more so for such individuals with dyslexia.

Summary

The optometrist can comanage cases of either general or specific RD and treat the vision-related problems. Appropriate referrals should be made to allied health and educational specialists. Screening for dyslexia, and possibly further testing, should be done by the optometrist when indicated from case history. One of the trends in education, the whole-language approach, is often inappropriate and inadequate for many students, especially dyslexic individuals. Other possible pitfalls in educational trends are the tendency of inappropriate referrals in cases of ADHD and a rush toward full inclusion of students with RD in regular classrooms, where they may not receive adequate instruction for their needs.

References

1. Christenson GN, Griffin JR, Wesson MD. Optometry's role in reading disabilities: resolving the controversy. J Am Optom Assoc 1990;61:363–72.

2. Wesson MD. Diagnosis and management of reading dysfunction for the primary care optometrist. Optom Vis Sci 1993;70:357–68.
3. Griffin JR. Office testing for dyslexia. Curr Opin Ophthalmol 1992;3:111–6.
4. Griffin JR, Walton HN, Christenson GN. The Dyslexia Screener (TDS). Culver City, CA: Reading and Perception Therapy Center, 1988.
5. Christenson GN, Griffin JR, De Land PN. Validity of the dyslexia screener. Optom Vis Sci 1991;68:275–81.
6. Guerin DW, Griffin JR, Gottfried AW, et al. Concurrent validity and screening efficiency of the dyslexia screener. Psychol Assessment 1993;5:369–73.
7. Griffin JR, Walton HN. Dyslexia Determination Test (DDT) (rev ed). Los Angeles: Instructional Materials and Equipment Distributors, 1987.
8. Wesson MD, Griffin JR, Christenson GN. Pre-Dyslexia Letter Coding Test (PLCT). Culver City, CA: Reading and Perception Therapy Center, 1991.
9. Griffin JR, Walton HN. Dyslexia Screener for First-Graders (DSF). Culver City, CA: Reading and Perception Therapy Center, 1990.
10. Griffin JR, Christenson GN, Walton HN. Adult Dyslexia Test (ADT). Culver City, CA: Reading and Perception Therapy Center, 1990.
11. Biberdorf DH, Petros TV, Olson K, et al. Examination of the validity of the Adult Dyslexia Test with college students. Presented at the annual meeting of the American Academy of Optometry, San Diego, Dec. 13, 1994.
12. Griffin JR, Walton HN, Lind YG. Spanish Screening Version of the DDT. Los Angeles: Instructional Materials and Equipment Distributors, 1989.
13. Griffin JR, Walton HN, Ward L. French (Canadian) Screening Version of the DDT, (Dépistage de Dyslexie: Version Québécoise). Culver City, CA: Reading and Perception Therapy Center, 1994.
14. Lemer P. Education for All Handicapped Children Act. J Behav Optom 1990;1:151–3.
15. Solan HA. Overview of Learning Disabilities. In MM Scheiman, MW Rouse (eds), Optometric Management of Learning-Related Vision Problems. St. Louis: Mosby, 1994;116.
16. Wilson BA. Thoughts on inclusion and multisensory structural language teaching. The Decoder (Millbury, MA) 1994;6:6.
17. Rosenthal JH. Hazy . . ., Crazy . . ., and/or Lazy?: The Maligning of Children with Learning Disabilities. San Rafael, CA: Academic Therapy, 1973.
18. Blachman BA. An Alternative Classroom Reading Program for Learning Disabled and Other Low-Achieving Children. In W Ellis (ed), Intimacy with Language: A Forgotten Basic in Teacher Education. Baltimore: Orton Dyslexia Society, 1987.
19. Golinkoff RM. Phonemic Awareness Skills and Reading Achievement. In FB Murray, JH Pikulski (eds), The Acquisition of Reading: Cognitive, Linguistic, and Perceptual Prerequisites. Baltimore: University Park Press, 1978.
20. Lundberg I, Olofsson A, Wall S. Reading and spelling skills in the first school years, predicted from phonemic awareness skills in kindergarten. Scand J Psychol 1980;21:159–73.
21. Mann VA. Longitudinal prediction and prevention of early reading difficulty. Ann Dyslexia 1984;34:117–36.
22. Routh DK, Fox B. Mm . . . Is a Little Bit of May: Phonemes, Reading, and Spelling. In KD Gadow, P Bialen (eds), Advances in Learning and Behavioral Disabilities, Vol 3. Greenwich, CT: JAI Press, 1984.

23. Stanovich KE. Explaining the variance in reading ability in terms of psychological processes: what have we learned? Ann Dyslexia 1985;35:67–96.
24. Vellutino FR, Scanlon D. Phonological coding and phonological awareness and reading ability: evidence from a longitudinal and experimental study. Merrill Palmer Q 1987;33:321–63.
25. Bradley L. Rhyme Recognition and Reading and Spelling in Young Children. In W Ellis (ed), Intimacy with Language: A Forgotten Basic in Teacher Education (2nd ed). Baltimore: Orton Dyslexia Society, 1988.
26. Content A, Kolinsky R, Morris J, Bertelson P, et al. Phonetic segmentation in prereaders: effect of corrective information. J Exp Child Psychol 1986;42:49–72.
27. Ball EW, Blachman BA. Phoneme segmentation training: effect on reading readiness. Ann Dyslexia 1988;38:208–25.
28. Lundberg I, Frost J, Petersen O. Effects of an extensive program for stimulating phonological awareness in preschool children. Reading Res Q 1988;23:263–84.
29. Olofsson A, Lundberg I. Can phonemic awareness be trained in kindergarten? Scand J Psychol 1983;24:35–44.
30. Solan HA, Mozlin R. The correlations of perceptual-motor maturation to readiness and reading in kindergarten and the primary grades. J Am Optom Assoc 1986;57:28–35.
31. Meares O. Figure/ground, brightness contrast and reading disabilities. Visible Lang 1980;14:13–29.
32. Irlen H. Successful treatment of learning disabilities. Paper presented to the 91st Annual Convention of the American Psychological Association. Anaheim, CA, 1983.
33. Fitzgerald BA. Tinted lens and dyslexia: a review of the literature. Aust Orthoptic J 1989;25:1–6.
34. Rosner J, Rosner J. The Irlen treatment: a review of the literature. Optician 1987;194:26–33.
35. Whiting PR. How difficult can reading be? Paper distributed by the Sydney College of Advanced Education, Australia, 1985.
36. Robson GL, Miles J. The use of coloured overlays to improve visual processing: a preliminary survey. Except Child 1987;34:65–70.
37. Cheetham JS, Ovenden JA. Tinted lenses; hoax or help? Aust J Remedial Educ 1987;19:10–1.
38. Stanley G. Coloured filters and dyslexia. Aust J Remedial Educ 1987;19:8–9.
39. O'Connor PD, Sofo F. Dyslexia and tinted lenses. A response to Gordon Stanley. Aust J Remedial Educ 1988;20:10–2.
40. Wilsher CR, Taylor JA. Commentary, tinted lenses and dyslexia. J Res Reading 1988;11:50–2.
41. Gole GA, Dibden SN, Pearson CC, et al. SPELD (SA) Tinted Lens Study Group (1989). Tinted lenses and dyslexics: a controlled study. Aust N Z J Ophthalmol 1989;17:137–41.
42. Cardinal DN, Griffin JR, Christenson GN. Do tinted lenses really help students with reading disabilities? Intervention School Clin 1993;28:275–9.
43. Fitzgerald BA. Effect of tinted lenses on contrast sensitivity in normal and dyslexic children. Master's thesis, University of Sydney, Australia, 1989: Appendix III, pp. xiv–xxix.

44. Cline D, Hofstetter HW, Griffin JR (eds). Dictonary of Visual Science (4th ed). Radnor, PA: Chilton, 1989.
45. Scheiman B, Blaskey P, Ciner EB, et al. Vision characteristics of individuals identified as Irlen filter candidates. Am Optom Assoc 1990;61:600–5.
46. Blaskey P, Scheiman M, Parisi M, et al. The effectiveness of Irlen filters for improving reading performance: a pilot study. J Learn Disabil 1990;23:604–12.
47. The 1986/87 Future of Visual Development/Performance Task Force. Special Report. The efficacy of optometric vision therapy. Am Optom Assoc 1988;59:95–105.
48. Denckla MB. Clinical syndromes in learning disabilities: the case for "splitting" vs. "lumping." J Learn Disabil 1972;5:401–6.

Appendix: Suppliers of Tests and Training Materials

Academic Therapy Publishers, 20 Commercial Blvd, Novato, CA 94949.
    Boder Test of Reading and Spelling Patterns
    Materials for phonetic training
    Wold Sentence Copy Test
Bernell Corporation, 750 Lincolnway East, P.O. Box 4637, South Bend, IN 46634.
    Aperture-Rule Trainer
    Bar Readers, Vectographic and Anaglyphic
    Brock String and Beads
    Computer Programs (including take-home software)
    Developmental Eye Movement Test (DEM)
    Dual Polachrome Illuminated Trainer
    Dyslexia testing materials such as the DDT and TDS
    Hart Chart
    Lens flippers and prism flippers
    SO/V9 Acuity Suppression Slide
    Vectograms and Tranaglyphs
    Miscellaneous testing and training materials
Christenson Therapy Center, 347 East La Salle Ave., Barron, WI 54812.
    Home Dyslexia Screening Test (HDST)
Creative Therapeutics, 155 Country Road, Cresskill, NJ 07626.
    Gardner Reversals Frequency Test
Efficient Seeing Publications, 7510 Soquel Dr., Box 28, Aptos, CA 95003.
    Alphabet Pencils
Growth Strategies, Inc., 3400 Canary St., #6, Appleton, WI 54915.
    Golf Visualization
    Metronome
    Vectograms and other testing and training materials

Instructional Materials and Equipment Distributors, 1520 Cotner Ave., Los Angeles, CA 90025.
    Dyslexia Determination Test (DDT)
    Spanish Screening Version of the DDT
    Therapy in Dyslexia and Reading Problems
    Various educational programs (e.g., Selma Herr Phonics)
Keystone View, Division of Mast/Keystone Inc., 4673 Aircenter Circle, Reno, NV 89502.
    Colored Circles (Lifesavers)
    Eccentric Circles
    VT Playing Cards (Sherman)
Learning Frontiers, Inc., 190 Admiral Cochran Dr., Suite 180, Annapolis, MD 21401.
    Opti-Mum Computer Programs (Ludlam)
MKM Materials, 809 Kansas City St., Rapid City, SD 57701.
    MKM Series (phonetic-visual training)
Modern Curriculum Press, 4350 Equity Dr., P.O. Box 2649, Columbus, OH 43216.
    Developmental Test of Visual-Motor Integration (VMI)
PRO-ED, 8700 Shoal Creek Blvd., Austin, TX 78757.
    Developmental Test of Visual-Motor Integration (VMI) and other
        materials for testing and therapy
Psychological and Educational Publications, 1477 Rollins Road, Burlingame, CA 94010.
    Test of Visual Perceptual Skills (TVPS)
    Test of Visual Perceptual Skills (TVPS) Upper Level
    Test of Auditory-Perceptual Skills (TAPS)
R.C. Instruments, 1578 Eastport Court, P.O. Box 109, Cicero, IN 46034.
    Computer Orthoptics (Cooper)
Reading and Perception Therapy Center, 3840 Main St., Culver City, CA 90232.
    Adult Dyslexia Test (ADT)
    Dyslexia Determination Test (DDT)
    Dyslexia Screener for First-graders (DSF)
    French DDT Test (Test de Dyslexie)
    French TDS Version (Depistage de Dyslexie)
    Home Dyslexia Screening Test (HDST)
    Predyslexia Letter Coding Test (PLCT)
    Spanish Screening Version of the DDT
    The Dyslexia Screener (TDS)
    Therapy in Dyslexia and Reading Problems
Recording for the Blind and Dyslexic, 20 Roszel Road, Princeton, NJ 08540.
    Tape recordings of books and academic material
Stereo Optical Co., Inc., 3539 N. Kenton Ave., Chicago, IL 60641.
    Vectograms
    Various tests and training equipment

Universal Attention Disorders, Inc., 4281 Katella Ave., Suite 215, Los Alamitos, CA 90720.

Test of Variables Attention (TOVA)

Vision Analysis, 136 Hillcroft Way, Walnut Creek, CA 94596.

Disparometer (Sheedy)

Vision Extension of the Optometric Extension Program Foundation, Inc., 1921 E. Carnegie Ave., Suite 3-L, Santa Ana, CA 92705. (Sample listing of available testing and training materials)

Accommodative flipper lenses

Adult Dyslexia Test (ADT)

Birch-Belmont, Auditory-Visual Integration Test (AVIT)

Computerized vision therapy programs

Developmental Test of Visual-Motor Integration (VMI)

Dyslexia tests (e.g., DDT, TDS, DSF)

Fixation Beads and String (Brock String)

Hidden Picture Games

Ideal Forms (VMI training)

Lifesaver Cards (Hendrickson fusion training)

Metronome (electronic)

Monroe Visual III Test. In R Lowry. Handbook of Diagnostic Tests for the Developmental Optometrist, 1970.

Stereopsis tests

Tachistoscopes

Test of Auditory Analysis Skills (Rosner TAAS)

Test of Visual Analysis Skills (Rosner TVAS)

Test of Visual Perceptual Skills (TVPS) Ages 4–12

Test of Visual Perceptual Skills (TVPS) Upper Level

Vectograms for binocular training

Wesson Fixation Disparity Card

Walker and Company, 720 Fifth Ave., New York, NY 10019.

Helping Children Overcome Learning Difficulties, by Jerome Rosner

Wayne Engineering, 1825 Willow Road, Northfield, IL 60093.

Afterimage strobe flasher

Perceptuomotor (talking) pen

Saccadic Fixator

Note: Many vision training devices, if not commercially and readily available, can be custom-made (e.g., letter reversal sheets for directionality training and sequential beads on a string for visual-sequential-memory training).

Index

Academic Therapy Publishers, 241
Accommodation therapy, 176–177
  lens flipper rock, 177
  near-far rock, 176–177
  steps in, 176
Accommodative accuracy, 123–125
Accommodative dysfunctions, 21, 78
Accommodative facility, 122–123
Accommodative skills, testing, 122–125
Accommodative sufficiency, 125
ADD. *See* Attention-deficit disorder (ADD)
Adenoidectomy, 112–113
ADHD. *See* Attention-deficit hyperactivity disorder (ADHD)
ADT, 148, 208
Adult Dyslexia Test (ADT), 148, 208
Agnosia, finger, 24
Alexia, 22
Allocation of attention, 102–103
Amacrine cell (AMA), 45, 46
Amblyopia, 40
Ametropia, 42, 123, 125
Aniseikonia, 78
Anisometropia, 21, 78
APD. *See* Auditory-perceptual deficit (APD)
Aperture-Rule Trainer (ART), 180–181
Arabic decimal system, 13
Asthenopia, 78
Astigmatism, 22
  hyperopic, 5
Attention-deficit disorder (ADD), 6, 24, 169
  auditory-perceptual deficit (APD) and, 113–114
  characteristics/symptoms, 113–114

Attention-deficit hyperactivity disorder (ADHD), 5, 113, 169, 211
  characteristics/symptoms, 113–114
Auditory discrimination, 108, 141–142
Auditory dyslexia. *See* Dysphonesia
Auditory figure-ground perception, 108
Auditory input, 108
Auditory integration, 108–109
Auditory lag, 108
Auditory localization, 108
Auditory memory, 109
Auditory output, 109
Auditory perception, 107–116
  categories, 108–109
    input, 108
    integration, 108–109
    memory, 109
    output, 109
  definition/description, 107–108
Auditory-perceptual deficit (APD), 108
  chronic otitis media and, 109–113
  attention-deficit disorder (ADD) and, 113–114
Auditory-perceptual matching, 109
Auditory-perceptual skills testing, 140-142
  auditory discrimination, 141–142
  auditory-visual integration, 140–141
Auditory-visual integration, 140–141
Auditory-Visual Integration Test, 125
Auditory-visual integration therapy, 198–200
  clap patterns, 199–200
  computerized games, 200
  Morse code, 200–201
  steps in, 198–199

Backward masking, 56
Badcock, D., 59
Beery Developmental Test of VMI (BVMI),
    86–87, 125
Bernell Corporation, 241
Bilateral integration, 84, 130–131
Bilateral integration therapy, 184–185
    jumping jacks, 184
    steps in, 184
    windshield wipers, 184–185
Billing, G., 57
Binocular dysfunction, 78
Binocular lens rock, 121
Bipolar cells
    depolarizing, 44
    extrafoveal, 44
    invaginating, 44
    midget (MB), 44
    on-center response, 44
Bipolar personality, 5
Birch-Belmont Auditory-Visual Integration Test,
    86–87, 140–141
Blindness, 22
Blob system, 48
Boder Test of Reading-Spelling Patterns, 29,
    147, 148
Bologna, N.B., 64–66
Bowling, A., 59
Brain, 170–172
Brannan, J.R., 62, 64, 66–68
Breitmeyer model, 59
Brock string, 178–180
Brown, C., 56
BVMI, 86–87, 125

CAP, 107
CAPD, 107–108
Case studies
    adult with dyslexia and tinted glasses, 230–236
    dyseidesia, 219–223
    dysnemkinphoneidesia, 227–229
    dysphoneidesia, 223–227
    nondyslexia with reading dysfunction, 219
Central auditory processing (CAP), 107
Central auditory processing disorder (CAPD),
    107–108
Characteristic decoding, 24
Chiastopic fusion, 181–183
Christenson Therapy Center, 241
Chronic otitis media, 109–113
    description, 109
    effects on learning, 110–111
    medical treatment, 112
    prevalence among children, 111
    risk factors, 111

stages, 111–112
    surgical treatment, 112–113
Cognitive development, periods of, 80
Colliculus, superior, 47–48
Comprehension, 16–17
Computer Orthoptics, 193
Cone cells, 42–44
Consensus theory, 26
Contrast sensitivity unit (CSU), 45–46
Convergence, 178
Convergence insufficiency, 21
Cortical system, 170–172
Creative Therapeutics, 241
CSU, 45–46
Cuneiform, 15
Cylert, 211

DDT. See Dyslexia Determination Test (DDT)
De Lange function, 62
Decoding, 16–19, 149–151, 154, 158
    characteristic, 24
    eidetic, 18, 19, 24–25, 26, 88, 149,
        151–152, 154, 158
    phonetic, 18, 19, 24–25, 26, 88, 149, 151,
        154, 158
DEM, 102–103, 120–122
Depolarizing bipolar cells, 44
Developmental Eye Movement (DEM) test,
    102–103, 120–122
Developmental Test of Visual Motor Integration,
    138
Dexedrine, 211
Diplopia, 79
Directionality, 84, 131–134
Directionality therapy, 185–189
    directional arrows, 187–188
    floor map, 186–187
    letter recognition, 188–189
    number recognition, 188–189
    Simon Says, 186
    steps in, 186
Disparometer, 127, 128
Divergence, 178
Double vision, 78
Down syndrome, 79
DSF, 148, 208
Dual Polachrome Illuminated Trainer, 180
Dynamic overshoot, 98
Dynamic retinoscopy, 123
Dyseidesia, 27–30, 86, 88, 89, 104, 160–161
    case study on, 219–223
    prognosis guidelines, 207
    testing, 149–154
        decoding patterns, 149–151
        encoding patterns, 151–153